HYPNOBIRTHING®
The Mongan Method

*A natural approach to a safe,
easier, more comfortable birthing*

Third Edition
MARIE F. MONGAN, M.Ed., M.Hy.

SOUVENIR PRESS

Note

The HypnoBirthing method and this book describing its techniques are not intended to represent a medically and anatomically precise overview of pregnancy and birthing, nor are they designed to represent medical advice or a prescription for medical procedure. The content of this book is not intended to replace the advice of a medical doctor. It is advisable for any pregnant woman to seek the advice of a medical doctor or a health-care professional before undertaking any pregnancy or labour-related programme.

Persons following any course of action recommended in this book or in the HypnoBirthing programme do so of their own free will. The author, the publisher, and the HypnoBirthing Institute assume no responsibility for any possible complication related to either the pregnancy or the labour of the participant.

To my daughter Maura,
whose decision to have a child gave me
the inspiration to recreate the programme of natural birthing
through which she was born in 1959 – a programme
that has been waiting these many years to come into being.
I salute her choice with loving gratitude.

To our several HypnoBirthing grandbabies
who were born since the inception of the programme:
Kyle Patrick, born January 3, 1990;
Jennifer Marie, born December 4, 1991;
Patrick John, born September 11, 1992;
Jessica Michelle, born March 27, 1993;
Meghan Taylor, born September 28, 1996;
Melissa Kelley, born November 25, 1996;
Rachel Katherine, born October 18, 1998;
Lurena Kelly, born April 17, 1999;
Garrison Forest, born September 9, 2000;
Jamie Madisyn, born May 12, 2001;
Shane Christopher, born June 26, 2002.

To my husband, Gene, always my patient labour companion
through the birth of each revision of this HypnoBirthing book.
Without his love and support, this book would not
have been birthed, expanded and rewritten.

If we hope to create
a non-violent world
where respect and kindness
replace fear and hatred …

We must begin with how
we treat each other
at the beginning of life

For that is where
our deepest patterns are set.

From these roots
grow fear and alienation …
– or love and trust.

SUZANNE ARMS, AUTHOR
Immaculate Deception
Immaculate Deception II

CONTENTS

ACKNOWLEDGMENTS

It is with the very deepest appreciation that I acknowledge:

The late Dr. Jonathan Dye of Buffalo, New York, an early pioneer in natural childbirth, who in the late 1800s, in his book, *Easier Childbirth,* espoused the philosophy upon which this programme is based – that birth is normal, natural and healthy, and, therefore, can be achieved "without pain or peril".

The late Dr. Grantly Dick-Read, 1890–1959, a husband, father, philosopher and Englishman, who, through his work in obstetrics and his book, *Childbirth Without Fear,* returned to women their rightful gift of truly natural childbirth. He is a prophet whose time is yet to come. His theories and the work he did to forward natural childbirth are the inspiration for this programme.

Those several couples who, at the very inception of HypnoBirthing, had complete belief in this programme and were willing to place their faith in the HypnoBirthing philosophy, confident that this most natural birthing method would provide for them the fulfillment they were seeking as they experienced the greatest celebration of life – childbirth. It's because of them and the trail they blazed for others to follow that HypnoBirthing has gained the recognition that it enjoys today.

Mary Ann Murphy, dear friend, who put the natural simplicity of the HypnoBirthing philosophy into form in her creation of our first logo depicting the love and family bonding that takes place during HypnoBirthing.

George Ferren, my right arm, without whom much of the day-to-day work of the HypnoBirthing Institute over these many years could never have been accomplished. He continues to be a mainstay in the growth and smooth running of the Institute.

FOREWORD

Marie Mongan is a woman who has devoted her entire life to working with women of all ages and in all walks of life. Through her book and the HypnoBirthing Method, she shares the conviction of her own personal birthing experience and her sensitivity to the emotional and spiritual needs of birthing women. The message about the normalcy of birth that this book delivers is an essential one for all families who believe in and care about birthing their babies in safety, calm and peace.

This book, and the HypnoBirthing programme itself, has provided me, and other doctors who share a belief in normal birth, a framework within which to practise obstetrics in the manner in which our education has qualified us and in the direction in which our hearts have led us. It has changed the way many of us practise obstetrics.

I began "delivering" babies in 1983. I believed in the use of drugs to manage obstetrical pain. In spite of my best efforts to use good sound medical judgment, I saw lots of complications, including babies with compromised breathing. I believed that epidurals were a medical blessing for labouring mothers. I had a 25 per cent C-section rate.

Many patients demanded natural births. I then performed hundreds of deliveries using pushing and blowing while holding off analgesics until the mother could no longer take the pain. I saw babies that were no longer respiratorily compromised, but both mother and baby was exhausted, and quite often there was a need for respiratory support with oxygen. But my C-section rate had fallen to 5 per cent.

Next, I used visualization and guided imagery with patients to manage pain. On occasion, I still had to use narcotics and a rare epidural. I continued to see exhausted babies who were not fully able to bond. I still had a C-section rate of 5 per cent.

Eventually, I began using hypnosis to manage pain during birth.

The results were okay. Babies were less often compromised and very rarely needed oxygen, but mothers still experienced painful births. My C-section rate remained at 5 per cent.

A few years ago, I made the transition to HypnoBirthing, and I now truly believe that normal birthing does not have to involve pain. I have attended over 200 births of women who prepared for birth by learning and using the techniques and philosophy of HypnoBirthing – "The Mongan Method". All of the families have left their birthings excited about the birth event. I see support people meaningfully involved with the mother and assisting in many different ways. I have had no complications. No babies have needed oxygen or any support other than warming by mother's body. My C-section count is three – in as many years. I have given absolutely no analgesic drugs since I began using HypnoBirthing with mothers.

Over the years, I have come to realise that during a birthing, I no longer perform "deliveries"; I attend and observe as mothers birth their babies in calm and comfort, and birthing companions receive the babies as they emerge. It is as if my new role is to be present to witness the miracle of HypnoBirthing.

Now I enthusiastically lecture to medical groups on a regular basis about the merits of HypnoBirthing as a means of achieving easier, more comfortable births for labouring mothers. I am more than happy to talk to health-care professionals (or anyone else) about my experiences with truly natural birthing. I have a large number of happy HypnoBirthing families – mothers and fathers – who love to talk about their own birthing experiences.

In my present position as a faculty member of the Atlanta Family Medicine Residency Program in Atlanta, Georgia, I train medical residents to use HypnoBirthing as an option for the families they will serve.

I heartily recommend this book, and the well thought-out programme that it accompanies, for its contribution toward making the birth of our children a positive and gentle step on the way to a better world.

Lorne R. Campbell, Sr, M.D.
Clinical Assistant Professor of Family Medicine,
Mercer School of Medicine
Assistant Clinical Professor of Family Medicine,
University of Rochester and SUNY-Buffalo School of Medicine

INTRODUCTION

My dream is that every woman, everywhere, will know the joy of a truly safe, comfortable and satisfying birthing for herself and her baby.

MARIE F. MONGAN

Preparing to welcome a baby is a life-changing experience, not just through pregnancy and birth, but for the rest of your lives. HypnoBirthing offers a remarkably simple, relaxed approach to this most important transition, as you step into your role as parents and, together, become a family.

This edition of *HypnoBirthing: The Mongan Method is* an expanded version of my earlier books used by parents as they prepare for gentle birth. It is designed especially to serve the 95 per cent of families whose pregnancies fall into the normal, low- or no-risk categories. If you are part of this vast majority, HypnoBirthing will teach you techniques for relaxation and visualisation, along with physical exercises and a sound nutritional guide that will help you to ease through a happy, healthy pregnancy and childbirth.

If you have not fully embraced the concept of normal, natural birth as your choice, this book will provide an opportunity for you to explore its theories and learn more about how developing a calm approach to pregnancy and birth will enable you to prepare for a safer, easier, more comfortable and more joyful birthing.

Understanding the origin of many of the beliefs and myths surrounding birth that we, as a culture, have come to accept can assist you in making some of the decisions you will face in preparing for this most important time in your lives. This book will introduce you to ways in which you can connect with your pre-born baby and build a better understanding of your baby as a conscious little person, who is fully able to interact with you, even before birth. You can learn how to prepare your mind and your body in such a way that you will be able to achieve a happier birthing regardless of your present intent.

For those of you who have already determined that you are committed to bringing your baby into the world with HypnoBirthing, this book serves as a textbook, used in conjunction with the instruction you will receive in a series of HypnoBirthing childbirth education classes taught by certified practitioners affiliated with the HypnoBirthing Institute. This book outlines the philosophy and many of the techniques used by HypnoBirthing families. You will gain much information and insight from reading this book. However, the comprehensive instruction and discussions covering specific methods, scripts and demonstrations provided by your HypnoBirthing practitioner during classes, and even during your birthing, will prove to be invaluable.

The content of this programme is not intended to replace the advice and care of a health-care provider. You should always seek the advice of a qualified professional caregiver for all pregnancy-related matters.

For information on HypnoBirthing classes in your area or for practitioner certification workshops, please visit our website at *www.hypnobirthing.co.uk*

A MESSAGE TO PARENTS

TO THE MOTHER

Your journey into parenthood is one of the most amazing experiences that you will ever know. Choosing to explore HypnoBirthing will make the event all the more fulfilling.

Making this choice, however, is only one of many decisions you and your partner will make along this journey. It will be a very busy time for you, and many of the decisions are so important when you consider how they could impact your lives and that of your baby.

A key factor for many of these decisions is closely tied to how you look upon birth and how you regard your own role in this adventure into pregnancy, birthing and parenting. I hope the material in *HypnoBirthing* will help you and your birthing companion to sort through many of the important aspects of pregnancy and birth, and assist you in your role as parents. The programme is designed for you both, for your birth companion will play a vital role during your pregnancy and the birthing itself. You will attend classes together and actively take part in exercises and practise. If you detect a bit of hesitancy on the part of your partner, perhaps you will want to consider a secondary birthing companion for your labour and birthing. Both people will be welcome at your classes. But know that it's not unusual for a partner who was initially hesitant to absolutely blossom when he or she becomes involved with the discussions that take place. Most become more willing to assume an active role through the preparation phases and labour, even if this wasn't the case at the beginning. You may also arrange for your HypnoBirthing practitioner to attend your birth. Many are professionally trained in labour support and are happy to attend.

The realisation that you are carrying and will soon give birth to a new life is bound to evoke a number of feelings and emotions that you have never felt before. Like most parents-to-be, much of your thinking is given over to this little baby you are carrying and for whose birth you are preparing. This is very important. Reflect on how very special you are, as well as your feelings about the changes that are taking place as your baby develops.

This experience, no matter how many children you have, is unique to you and your baby. This child will never be physically born again, and its birth can never be duplicated. There are no other human beings in the world who could conceive this tiny person and bring him into the world. This is a once-in-a-lifetime event, and it's only natural that you and your birthing companion are seeking a birthing that is as safe, satisfying and naturally comfortable for your baby as possible.

HypnoBirthing is designed to enhance those feelings of uniqueness and awe, helping you to reach an awareness of your body as the most perfect instrument of nature – the vehicle through which your child will miraculously develop and enter into this world. Birthing is nature characterised at its best. It is the implementation of the highest power of life that ensures the survival of the human race. All other works of nature pale by comparison to the miracle of birth, and you both are at the heart of that wonderful miracle.

Nature has been working with you from the very beginning of your pregnancy to prepare your body for this great wonder. Your perfected body works in harmony with your mind. You will learn how to work with nature, and you will become consumed with preparing for a naturally safe birth through proper nutrition, good posture, fitness and an attitude of trust in the birthing process. You will come to understand that when your mind is free of fear and tension, your body can be free of pain and will function as it was created to do.

With these understandings and the HypnoBirthing techniques that you will practise, you empower yourself with confidence that will allow you to experience the birthing of your baby with relaxed expectation and joy.

TO THE FATHER OR BIRTH COMPANION

You who look forward to serving as a birthing companion – husband, partner, friend, sister, mother – have a very special part to play in HypnoBirthing. Countless women who have given birth through this programme have laid the success of their birthing experience directly upon the support and assistance of the birth companion. The support and bonding that take place throughout labour and birthing create a partnership, the beauty of which defies description. Couples report that they become closer than they ever thought they could be. The knowledge that she is supported by a caring and loving companion is one of the most important factors in maintaining the emotional well-being of the pregnant mother and the baby she is carrying.

It is important that you share in the task of selecting a health-care provider who will support you in your wishes to have a normal, safe birth. Most dads find that they are quite welcome when they attend prenatal visits and enjoy sharing the excitement of learning about their baby's growth and development. Your willingness to take the lead in assuring that the birthing you both have planned becomes a reality is vital, and your confidence will help to build the mother's confidence, as well as pave the way for a good relationship with your provider.

By learning techniques to support the mother during pregnancy, and participating in the necessary practise at home, you give assurance to your baby that he or she is already an important part of your lives.

As an integral part of the process, you bring the necessary elements of trust and assurance to the birthing environment. You will be the facilitator – helping her to condition her mind to relax in response to your prompts. The sound of your voice and the touch of your hand will guide her through labour. The attention, understanding, encouragement and closeness creates a sharing that is unequalled, and all these things will help create a bond that will linger throughout your lives.

You may feel unsure about your role in the birthing room at first. This is natural. As you guide the mother with your prompts during labour, however, you'll quickly sense the importance of giving this kind of support, continuously assuring her of her ability to birth gently and to maintain the peace and calm that surround the birth. Working with her through each uterine surge, you will become fully consumed in her responsiveness, and any awareness of others will totally dissipate. You will instinctively know what you must do, and you will become oblivious to the coming and going of caregivers.

If you are approaching this birth with fear of watching someone you love experience discomfort, the HypnoBirthing classes will allay those fears. You and the birthing mother will learn techniques that will alleviate discomfort and possibly even eliminate it. Your support and love help to make this happen.

A woman in labour can be vulnerable, sensitive and unassertive. You will be her advocate, her spokesperson, her guide. You will be the liaison between her and your caregivers, both before and during birthing. Your involvement in preparing the Birth Preference Sheets and in speaking for the two of you to ensure that the plan is carried out will be among your most important tasks. Your presence and support, especially during the actual birthing, cannot be equalled. And, at the moment of birth, you will feel the exhilaration that comes with knowing that together you have made this miracle – one that neither of you will ever forget.

> Somebody said that no one
> can love a child the way a mother can.
> Somebody was never a father.

AUTHOR UNKNOWN

The Birth of Natural Childbirth

> It is not only that we want to bring about an easy labour,
> without risking injury to the mother or the child; we must
> go further. We must understand that childbirth is
> fundamentally a spiritual, as well as a physical,
> achievement. ... The birth of a child is the ultimate
> perfection of human love.
>
> GRANTLY DICK-READ, 1953

HypnoBirthing's philosophy is tied to the way that birthing was practiced in ancient times – as a celebration of life. Its practical origin lies in the work of men of modern science, particularly in the theories of an early twentieth-century English obstetrician named Dr. Grantly Dick-Read.

Dr. Dick-Read first became sensitive to the true nature of labour and birth in a humble, poverty-ridden setting in London in 1913. As a young intern in London's Whitechapel District in the heart of the East End slums, he was called to attend a woman in labour. After travelling on his bicycle through mud and rain, he arrived about three in the morning at a low hovel near some railway arches. He found his way to a small apartment where he discovered his patient in a dim room, soaked from the rain pouring in from the leaky roof. She was covered only with sacks and an old black skirt. He asked permission to put the mask over her face and administer chloroform. Her emphatic refusal was a first for Dick-Read. He returned the chloroform and mask to his bag, stood back and watched as she, with little more than gentle breathing, birthed her baby. The baby was born with no fuss or noise from the mother. As he prepared to leave, Dick-Read asked why she had refused the relief from pain.

She gave him an answer that he was never to forget. "It didn't hurt. It wasn't supposed to, was it, Doctor?" This honest answer, given in a deep cockney accent, has had a profound effect on birthing for many decades.

When he returned to the hospital that morning, Dick-Read was surprised to hear the nurse explain that it was a very boring night, but that things might pick up because the woman in Room 308 might be having some trouble. He had heard those words before, but now it was not something he could easily dismiss. Unless there was a problem, birth was considered boring?

In the months that followed, he sat night after night with educated, very affluent women in the London hospital. He watched the agony and terror that they experienced, and his mind kept drifting back to the woman in the hovel under the railway tracks. He mentally compared his present patients with the tranquil, comfortable woman who birthed with no difficulty, and he asked, "Why?"

Similar experiences presented themselves to Dick-Read when he was in the service during World War I. On a battlefield in a foreign land, a woman, very much in labour, approached a trench asking for the field doctor. She was directed to Grantly Dick-Read, and they helped her down into the trench. She seemed to ignore Dick-Read and proceeded to give birth, very easily and apparently with no discomfort, just as the woman had on that evening in London. The woman in the trench seemed oblivious to the war that was going on around her. When she had birthed her baby, she wrapped it, received help to leave the trench, and went on her way once more across the battlefield.

On another occasion he encountered a labouring woman, propped against an embankment, giving birth. The baby arrived easily. He watched as she waited for some time, holding the baby in her arms. He could see that the umbilicus had begun to thin, like a string. Having completed her task, she started her journey back to her village, her newborn in her arms. Once more he had witnessed a normal birth. There was nothing wrong with her labour.

These events prompted Dick-Read to question his belief about what he had been taught about labour. He puzzled over what these simple women brought to their birthings that allowed them to birth their babies without the usual histrionics that he was accustomed to seeing from more sophisticated women. Over time, it became clear to him that the answer lay, not in what these simple women brought to their labours, but rather what they didn't bring – fear.

With these experiences behind him, he embarked upon several years of study. From this study came his theory that when fear is not present, pain is not present. Fear causes the arteries leading to the uterus to constrict and become tense, creating pain. In the absence of fear, the muscles relax and become pliable, and the cervix is able to naturally thin and open as the body pulsates rhythmically and expels the baby with ease.

Sometime during the 1920s, Dick-Read forwarded a paper spelling out the answer to the question, "What's wrong with labour?" He called his theory the "Fear–Tension–Pain Syndrome" and offered a primary premise that fear is the cause of tension within the body, and in particular in the uterus, and that tension inhibits the natural birthing process, prolonging labour and causing pain. His colleagues thought he was mad to even entertain the notion that birth can be pain free, and no one would listen. His theory later gained some attention with the publication of his book, *Natural Childbirth*, in 1933, further setting down his ideas and stating that the body is, in fact, perfectly equipped to decrease the discomfort of birth. His colleagues, accustomed to "conducting deliveries" with drugs and forceps, still turned a deaf ear. The theory that something within our own bodies that, in the absence of fear and tension, releases a natural relaxant that facilitates easy birth was too radical for the time.

ENDORPHINS – THE BODY'S NATURAL PAINKILLERS

Dick-Read was more than a half century ahead of his time. He couldn't put a name to it, but he knew from observation that when labouring mothers are not limited by fear, something wonderful happens that permits easier birth. The body fills with its own natural relaxant.

Scientists have long searched for alternatives to painkilling drugs, but it wasn't until the mid-seventies that it was discovered that a source of natural analgesic lies within the body itself. Studying the way in which opiates work upon the body, American researchers discovered that opiate molecules, locking onto special receptor sites of neurons in the central nervous system, slowed down the firing rate of the neurons. They found that if they decreased the firing rate of the neurons, it resulted in a decrease in the sensation of pain. A state of calm was the missing ingredient that made the decrease possible.

With this information behind them, it was not long before scientists isolated **endorphins** – neuropeptides in the brain and pituitary gland that have an effect 200 times that of morphine. Endorphins produce a tranquil amnesiac condition. The discovery validated Dick-Read's suspicions.

This amnesiac condition occurs naturally in birth in all mammals as the labouring mother nears the end of the opening phase of her labour. That dreaded period, referred to by other methods as "transition", naturally disappears as she slips into a tranquil state, goes deeper within to her baby and her birthing body, leaving all the distractions of the rest of the world behind as she and her baby connect and give birth.

In the mid-fifties, the second printing of Dick-Read's book, *Revelations on Childbirth,* was published in the United States under the title *Childbirth Without Fear.* For those of us who didn't buy into the generally accepted belief that there is something terribly wrong with labour, he became our hero. We were listening, and many women of my generation experienced absolutely wonderful births.

Dick-Read's teachings became the foundation for two important American birthing movements in the twentieth century: the Lamaze Method and Husband-Coached Childbirth, known more commonly today as the Bradley Method. For over a decade, women were able to birth their babies free of pain with the Lamaze Method. Unfortunately, the medical establishment co-opted the course content, and the Lamaze philosophy was undermined. Many instructors added their own spin, or that of the facility employing them, to the original work, and eventually the Lamaze name was replaced with "Prepared Childbirth" classes. In recent years the programme has begun to recapture much of the original intent of its founder, Ferdinand Lamaze.

In 1989, the HypnoBirthing movement came onto the birthing scene, bringing with it a return to the belief that every woman has within her the power to call upon her natural maternal instinct to birth her babies in joy and comfort in a manner that most mirrors nature.

> My theories are drawn from observation at the bedside of labouring mothers, not in a laboratory.
>
> DR. GRANTLY DICK-READ

The Birth of HypnoBirthing

In June 1954, I was twenty-one years old and sure that the world was mine for the taking. On the fifth, I graduated from a small teachers' college in Plymouth, New Hampshire. I had already signed a contract to teach in the autumn, and now, with degree in hand, I was realising the fruition of a childhood dream: I was going to be a teacher.

One week later, I was married. It was a fairy-tale wedding between high school sweethearts. I was assuming two new, life-changing roles at the same time, but why not?

I began teaching in September and knew that I had found the niche that would be mine for the rest of my life. My husband was discharged from the service in late autumn of that year, and we began our lives together in a small lumber town in the foothills of New Hampshire's White Mountains.

In January, I missed a period. I was sure it was the result of the bronchitis that had attacked me in December. I couldn't be pregnant.

Anxious to get my system back on schedule, I made an appointment with my family doctor. When we sat in his office after my examination, his diagnosis sent me into a state of shock. I was pregnant.

Neither of us had even considered having a child at that point in our lives. My husband had enrolled in college under the GI Bill; I was very involved in lesson plans and adjusting to all of the experiences that come with being a first-year teacher. Our marriage was so new that we hadn't even finished furnishing the small, one-bedroom apartment that we were renting. I wasn't sick in the morning, I didn't show any signs of bloating, and my appetite hadn't taken any bizarre twists. We just couldn't be having a baby now. Not now!

For several days I was tempted to go back to the doctor and insist that it was simply my bronchitis that was still raising havoc with my body, and I really wasn't pregnant after all.

Then one morning I awakened feeling a strange, exciting glow about myself. There was a voice from deep inside me that kept repeating, "I'm going to have a baby". I felt an exhilaration that was different from anything I have ever felt before, and I liked it. I don't know where it came from, but from that moment I became enthralled with the wonderment of what was happening inside me. I became consumed with thoughts of my pregnancy and our new baby.

I decided that this was not going to be a "usual pregnancy", complete with aching back, swollen feet or any of the other complaints common to pregnancy. My birthing was not going to be one of drugged compliance with no recollection of the experience. The premise that birthing, by nature, had to be a painful ordeal was totally unacceptable to me. I could not believe that a God who had created the body with such perfection could have designed a system of procreation that was flawed. So many questions prevented me from accepting the concept of pain in birthing. Why are the two sets of muscles of the uterus the only muscles that do not perform well under normal conditions? Why are the lesser animals blessed with smooth, easy birthing while we, the very highest of creatures, made in the image and likeness of God, are destined to suffer? And why are women in some cultures able to have gentle, comfortable births? Are we women in the Western world less loved, less indulged, less blessed than they? It didn't make sense to me logically or physiologically.

Even more importantly, I could not believe that a loving God would commit so cruel a hoax as to make us sexual beings so that we would come together in love to conceive and then make the means through which we would birth our children so excruciatingly painful.

I read everything I could get my hands on in an attempt to support my belief that pain is inappropriate in the course of uncomplicated birthing. I summarily dismissed most of what I picked up. All of the literature of the time was laden with medical "what ifs". The focus was on all that could go wrong in labour. I was discouraged.

Then I remembered an article in *Life* magazine that I had read when I was in high school. It told of a woman who birthed naturally in the Grace–New Haven Hospital in Connecticut. I knew if I could find that magazine, I could find the support for my beliefs, and I could track down the name of the English doctor whose method of natural childbirth the hospital had adopted. I found the magazine at our local library and subsequently found Dr. Grantly Dick-Read's book, *Childbirth Without Fear*. I knew immediately that this concept was the answer to the drug-free, painless and safe birthing I was seeking for myself and especially for our baby. One didn't hear much about baby's safety or comfort at that time. It was all about the mother's experience, but nothing about how she and her partner viewed the experience or their hopes and dreams for the birthing. The idea of family didn't enter into birthing considerations.

I discarded all of the negative literature devoted to descriptions of labouring mothers trying to cope with and survive the "excruciating pain of childbirth", and focused on Dick-Read's theory of eliminating the Fear–Tension–Pain Syndrome. I was excited and looked forward to my normal, natural birth, awake, alert, and free of the fear and pain that it caused. I was also excited to learn that the doctors at Grace were in agreement that fear of pain could actually create real pain in labour. They wholly accepted the concept that "mental fears are translated into physical tensions that produce needless pain". They generally conceded that most births – though not all – are uncomplicated and could be accomplished with a minimum of drugs, artificial aid and intervention. I liked what I read.

I was prepared for natural birthing, but not for the reaction of other people from both within and outside of the medical field. No one thought I was serious about having a baby without taking anaesthesia. Friends laughed at me for suggesting that it was possible to have a baby naturally at a time when all women were "knocked out" with general anaesthesia. I was ridiculed and insulted by anaesthesiologists, who were just introducing the "caudal", a type of spinal block that required that the birthing mother lie absolutely flat for hours after she birthed to avoid recurring headaches that could be a problem for years to come. Luckily, my husband and my family, accustomed to my propensity for doing the unusual, provided sceptical support.

When I arrived at the hospital in labour, I explained that I was going to have a natural birth. Smirks appeared on the nurses' faces immediately. Shortly after I was "prepped" for labour with a pubic shave and an enema, a nurse kindly reassured me, "When the pains get unbearable, you can have a shot of Demerol to ease them". I was mocked when I declined the offer and was left alone in a dark labour room, listening to the insufferable ticking of a "Baby Ben" clock that was placed by my bedside so that I could "time" my "labour pains". I was ignored by nurses who wouldn't accept that I was in advanced labour, and I was told that when I finally went down that hall to the delivery room that I would be "yelling and screaming like the rest of them".

A very short time later, I told the nurse that I was crowning. She reluctantly agreed to examine me and, indeed, the yelling began – but it was the nurses who were yelling, not I.

They pushed my legs together and insisted that I pant. I asked to be allowed to birth my baby there and then, but they rushed me, still holding my legs together and panting, to the delivery room. Once there, my wrists were strapped to the sides of the delivery table with leather straps, and my legs were tied into the stirrups that held my knees and legs four feet into the air. My head was held as the ether cone was forced onto my face. That was the last I remembered. I awakened sometime later, violently ill from the ether, and was informed that I had "delivered" a beautiful baby boy, whom I would be able to see in the morning. The nurse cautioned me not to be alarmed at the red bruises on his face from the forceps. "That's normal." My husband was allowed to visit me for ten minutes. Neither of us held or even saw our son Wayne that night.

When I did see my baby for the first time, I was horrified to think of what he must have experienced as he was being "yanked" into the world. I felt so let down, and I was terribly resentful. The natural birth I had planned for my baby had been stolen from me, and my baby had suffered needlessly. My husband saw our son only through the window of the nursery for the next five days, as no one was allowed to visit when "the babies are on the floor". Our family bonding was nonexistent.

Two years later when I was in labour with our second son, Brian, the course of my labour was as peaceful and comfortable as it had been with my first labour, but the birthing played out as before – it was a total blank. When I was finally allowed to see Brian at the "appointed time", I again found red blotches on my baby's face from the pressure of forceps. Five days later when we were discharged from the hospital, my husband was able to hold him for the first time. I was beside myself with anger. I had asked for nothing more than to be allowed to birth my baby in peace. I was not asking for any extras. There was no need for me to be anaesthetised, strapped and assaulted.

Very early in my third pregnancy, I approached my doctor and said, "I think we need to talk". He laughed and responded with a question.

"Talk? What do we need to talk about, Mickey? This is your third baby; you know how it's done."

With a smile that lasted through my entire sentence, I replied, "Yes, Doctor, but you don't".

The smile saved me. He was obviously shocked that a layperson could make such an accusation, smile or no smile, but he was a friend. He recovered and asked what I meant.

I saw my opening, and I took it. I told him how disappointed I was with the way my previous births were handled. I said that I felt betrayed when, in spite of his agreement to support me in my wish for a natural birth, he was not there to support me or intercede for me when it came time for me to birth. And so, with no one to tell them differently, the nursing staff faithfully carried out their routine of "preparing" me for birthing with restraints and ether. I repeated how important it was to me to birth my baby safely without drugs. I said that this time I was determined to birth naturally, even if it meant that I would have to travel elsewhere to find a caregiver who would hear my concerns for my baby and listen to my emotional needs as a birthing mother.

Few babies were born at home at that time, so I knew my only real option was to elicit the complete support of the right caregiver – hopefully, my own doctor. He assured me that he could be that person and asked what I wanted him to do.

I asked that this information be put onto my chart so everyone would know that I didn't want to be offered drugs and was not to be tied to the birthing table. He smiled, wrote notes on my record and asked if that would make me happy. I lowered my head and looked at him from under my brow and replied, "I'm not quite done yet".

He picked up his pen again and said, "Okay, what else?"

My reply was spoken very quickly because I didn't trust that the words would really come out if I hesitated. "I'd like my husband with me in the labour room and by my side in the delivery room."

To understand how outlandish this request was, you have to realise that in the late fifties husbands were not allowed beyond the lobby of most hospitals. There were no lounge areas conveniently located near the maternity ward where fathers could pace. Most were sent home to wait for the call that would tell them, "It's all over".

The doctor's pen flew across the desk. He bounced forward in his swivel chair and said, "Oh, come on now, you can't ask me to stick my neck out that far"!

I explained that I didn't want him to do anything that he didn't feel comfortable with. If he were not comfortable, I would understand and seek another provider. He thought for a moment and gave me the answer for which I was hoping. "Why not?"

I was ecstatic. I had his support and his promise to officially chart that I was to be accommodated in fulfilling what I believe was the original "birth plan". I trusted that this time he would come through for me, and he did. My husband was by my side throughout my two-hour labour, and he accompanied me to the delivery room and stood by my side while our daughter was born – a first for that hospital and the entire region.

My arms and legs were free, and anaesthesia was not used. I was awake and energised. My joy was unparalleled. Though I had laboured naturally before, I finally had my fully natural birth. Maura came into the world safely and undrugged. The only sad part was that neither of us was able to hold our baby and bond with her immediately. She was whisked out of the room and taken to the nursery for no apparent reason.

A few minutes later, I stood at the nursery window watching them bathe my daughter – this at a time when women were hardly allowed out of bed for at least a day or more after birthing. I felt as though I could just sweep her up in my arms and go home. But that was not to be the case. Confinement at that time was at least four days.

Everyone with me that evening was on a natural high. My doctor was so excited that he stayed up until three in the morning, reading everything he had available on Dr. Grantly Dick-Read's theory of natural childbirth. I was told that my birthing was the talk of the entire hospital for three shifts. Unfortunately, this fascination and curiosity was short-lived. Within days, my birthing was dismissed as a "fluke". I was told that some women have an incredible tolerance for pain, and, after all, my baby girl was only six pounds, three ounces. The trail I thought I had blazed was quickly swept over. Nothing changed.

My fourth birthing followed the same smooth path, although our son Shawn weighed in at eight pounds, three ounces – a full two pounds heavier than Maura. Minutes after I was brought back to my room, I found that, once again, I had to go to the nursery to get a glimpse of my baby. When they finished bathing, weighing and dressing Shawn, they wheeled the little bassinette over to the window. He was on one side of the glass; I was on the other. That was the extent of my bonding with my baby.

My doctor, still fascinated but not at all convinced, told me that he was unbelievably impressed that someone could endure that much pain so calmly and without anaesthesia. In spite of my frequent boasts of feeling nothing but tightening sensations, I was not successful in opening his mind to what natural birthing could be for the mothers who were to follow me. Leather straps, ether cones, spinals and stirrups were to prevail for women for years to come.

THE FIRST HYPNOBIRTHING

Through the years, I shuddered each time I heard a woman speak of being in horrific agony while having her baby. It saddened me because I knew that the pain could have been eased and, in many instances, even eliminated. I felt so helpless. Whenever I spoke of easier childbirth, my listeners looked at me with shock or polite dis-belief.

In 1987, I became certified in hypnotherapy for use in the coun-selling practice that I had maintained throughout the years that I was dean at a women's college and later in my role as the director of a business school for women. Being involved in hypnotherapy caused me to think back to my birthings. I realised for the first time that I had, indeed, used self-hypnosis to achieve the degree of relaxation that made it possible for me to experience painless childbirth. (Grantly Dick-Read emphatically denied that his method was at all connected with hypnosis. He felt that hypnosis brought women to a totally disassociated state that took them away from the birthing experience. With a better understanding of hypnosis today, we now know that a person in a hypnotic state is fully awake, is in an even heightened state of awareness and totally in control.) I was, indeed, in self-hypnosis when I laboured with my children.

A year or so after I became a hypnotherapist, my daughter, Maura, told me that she was going to have a baby. I was determined that she experience only the very best and most satisfying birthing possible. From my newly awakened interest in birthing came a childbirth education programme, combining the advantages of self-hypnosis with the knowledge of natural childbirth. I called the method "HypnoBirthing".

I began to make notes based on my own personal and professional experiences early in 1989. I delighted in the prospect of developing the programme that would allow Maura, who was the first baby in the area to be born with a method of self-hypnosis, to bring her own child into the world with HypnoBirthing. There were two other mums preparing for birthing using my method, and I prayed that Maura would be the first to birth. She was.

Maura didn't have the benefit of videos or success stories of the thousands of other women who had birthed their babies through HypnoBirthing, but she knew that she wanted to birth her baby safely and did what was necessary to achieve it. She talked with her midwife about the kind of birth she was seeking: gentle, natural and free of narcotics that could harm her baby. She won her midwife's support and encouragement and had an uneventful, healthy and happy pregnancy.

When she arrived at the hospital to birth, Maura was met by a curious, but totally supportive labour and birthing staff. During the five hours that she laboured, a continuous stream of nurses and midwives found one reason or another to peek into the room to find the source of the soft music and to observe this enigma – a birthing mother, deeply connected with her baby and her birthing body, who looked, for all the world, as though she were quietly resting. There were none of the usual signs of a woman who was nearing completion. I believe that, on a deeper level, Maura's own birth left an imprint in her subconscious of what birth should be. She fully trusted her body, and it worked for her.

On January 3, 1990, the first HypnoBirthing baby, our grandson Kyle, was born. We had gone full circle – from Maura, the first natural-birth baby in the region, to Kyle, the first HypnoBirthing baby. I can't even begin to express how moving this experience was for me.

The hospital personnel were in awe. They had seen women experience gentle birthing before, but they knew that this birth was not to be dismissed. What they were seeing was not a fluke, but a birth that had been carefully and lovingly planned, prepared for and achieved.

Since then, we have welcomed ten more HypnoBirthing grandbabies into our family. They are a wonderful group of particularly nice human beings, showing those special qualities that other HypnoBirthing parents from all over the world are telling us they see in their HypnoBirthing babies: gentleness, compassion, self-confidence and love.

HYPNOBIRTHING TODAY

I wasn't aware when I first developed HypnoBirthing that it would grow from a local phenomenon into an international movement. I didn't realise the extent to which birthing mothers around the world were clamouring for a birthing method that would allow them to birth their babies safely, without drugs, and to be able to do it in comfort. They are turning to HypnoBirthing to provide that means.

Each year, thousands of couples are joining the ranks of HypnoBirthing families. Like you, these couples want the very best for themselves and their children, and they are taking responsibility for seeing that it happens. They are planning and directing the course of their pregnancies, and confidently looking forward to a joyful birthing experience. Some, who already embrace the philosophy of gentle birth, are relieved to find that, in addition to offering their baby a safe birth, they also are able to achieve a comfortable birth.

HypnoBirthing is helping women reclaim their right to call upon their natural birthing instincts, and with the total involvement of their partners, they are creating one of the most memorable experiences of their lives.

Because of the growing acceptance of HypnoBirthing: The Mongan Method, gentle, comfortable birth is gradually making its way into the birthing rooms of many hospitals. Many leading hospitals throughout the country are teaching gentle birthing and offering HypnoBirthing instruction in their childbirth education classes. More families are deciding to birth in the comfort and privacy of their own homes, and some are utilising the advantages of underwater birthing in hospitals and at home. Those families who choose to birth in hospitals or birthing centres are finding a congenial and supportive atmosphere in which they can have their babies, naturally and calmly, creating joyful memories for themselves and their babies.

People within the medical field are becoming part of the sweeping HypnoBirthing movement. An increasing number of compassionate caregivers and birthing facility administrators are listening to the emotional and spiritual needs of parents and are accommodating those needs in hospitals, birth centres and homes in over twenty-two countries. They are comfortable with the notion that birth is about the birthing family and are not threatened at the thought of relinquishing the progression of birth to the parents they serve, while they attend in support. The large network of certified HypnoBirthing practitioners continues to grow as the demand for HypnoBirthing grows from families across the globe.

The concept of calm, uninterrupted birthing is now being met with far less scepticism. The countless telephone calls and testimonials we receive tell us that HypnoBirthing is succeeding in creating a shift in the view of birthing.

On the other hand, the harsh, demeaning, sometimes violent practices still in effect in many birthing facilities tell us that we cannot rest on our laurels. Our job is just beginning. Unnecessary interventions, including a growing number of needless inductions, augmentations and surgical births, are often imposed upon families who wish to birth naturally, even when there is no medical urgency. The birthing rooms of hospitals, though they give an appearance that might rival many five-star hotels, must be coupled with a shift in birthing philosophy from those who come to these settings to attend mothers in labour. Otherwise, we will continue to see many mothers birthing their babies while surrounded by machines and apparatus, hooked up to belts and tubes, looking more like scientific experiments than fulfilled and joyful birthing women.

HypnoBirthing continues to be a safe vehicle for those parents who are learning that they have options and are actively exploring them to find the optimal setting for their birthings. They are not willing to settle for anything less than the best for their babies.

Dr. Christiane Northrup, author of *Women's Bodies, Women's Wisdom*, sums it up well with this challenge to all birthing mothers:

Imagine what might happen if the majority of women emerged from their labour beds with a renewed sense of the strength and power of their bodies, and of their capacity for ecstasy through giving birth. When enough women realise that birth is a time of great opportunity to get in touch with their true power, and when they are willing to assume responsibility for this, we will reclaim the power of birth and help move technology where it belongs – in the women, not as their master.

Taking the Birthing World by Calm: The Philosophy of HypnoBirthing

> According to physiological law, all natural, normal functions
> of the body are achieved without peril or pain. Birth is a
> natural, normal physiological function for normal, healthy
> women and their healthy babies. It can, therefore, be
> inferred that healthy women, carrying healthy babies, can
> safely birth without peril or pain.
>
> DR. JONATHAN DYE, 1891

HypnoBirthing is as much a philosophy of birth as it is a technique
or method for birthing. The basic tenet of the programme is that
childbirth is a normal, natural and healthy function for women. As
such, birth can be accomplished gently and calmly for the very
large number of women who are not in a high-risk situation.

Like the bodies of our sister creatures in nature, the bodies of
healthy pregnant women instinctively know how to birth, just as
their bodies instinctively know how to conceive and how to nurture
the development of the babies they are carrying. HypnoBirthing
helps mothers align with their own innate capacity to be able to give
birth gently, comfortably, powerfully and joyfully. We don't promise births that are totally free of discomfort, but we firmly believe
that comfortable birthing is a possibility for 95 per cent of birthing
mothers through this philosophy and programme.

A HypnoBirthing mother learns to embrace her body's innate
knowledge of birthing, to relax into her birthing process, working
with her body and her baby. She trusts that each knows how to do
its job. She wants this experience to unfold naturally without interruption. In doing this, she eliminates fatigue and shortens her

birthing time. The result is a truly rewarding and satisfying birth experience, with the entire family, including the baby, being awake, alert and calm, yet energized.

This is not a new concept; women have been birthing this way for centuries. The efficacy of this method was recognised and recorded as early as the days of Hippocrates and Aristotle, who repeatedly wrote that nature is the best physician and that it should be allowed to function without the intrusion of "meddlesome interference". Birth was looked upon as a beautifully orchestrated natural function, designed to ensure the survival of the human race. There are many in medicine today who share this philosophy.

Dr. Michel Odent, world-renowned advocate of gentle birthing, points out, "One cannot help a physiological process. The point is not to hinder it". He advises that birth attendants keep their hands in their pockets when they are by the side of a birthing mother so that the natural process can play out.

HypnoBirthing recognises the importance of the role of the family in birthing, whether the family consists of a mother and her baby, a couple who are expecting their first baby, or a family who already has welcomed one or more children into their home. Accordingly, the birth companion – whether a father, a relative, a partner or a friend – plays an integral role in preparation for birth and in the actual birth experience.

The HypnoBirthing view of birth is that it is a natural extension of the sexuality of a man and a woman, and, therefore, we believe that birth is about them. It is about family fulfillment. It's about helping men to let go and free themselves from centuries-old programming that has gradually eroded their role in birth and made them onlookers in one of the greatest and most important experiences of their lives. It's about the manner in which they welcome a new little person into their family and into their lives, and it's about accepting responsibility for achieving the safest and most comfortable birth for their baby.

For the birthing parents, birth is not about science; it's not about anatomy; it's not about doctors or midwives or nurses; it's not about who has control. It's about family – parents and their babies.

Families embracing the belief that birth is about them and the wonderful life-changing transition they are making into parenthood don't really need to be taught *how* to birth. They simply need to learn *about* birth. They come to understand that when the mind is free of stress and fear that cause the body to respond with pain, nature is free to process birth in the same well-designed manner that it does for all other normal physiological functions.

In spite of the fact that today a large number of births still take place in a medical environment, HypnoBirthing practitioners believe birth is not a medical incident. An otherwise healthy pregnant woman is not diseased, and she is not ill. Her body is participating in the most amazing function of nature – childbirth.

HypnoBirthing is a collaborative method of childbirth, not an alternative method. The programme philosophy does not preclude the introduction of medical intervention, per se. It precludes the introduction of routine, arbitrary or unnecessary medical intervention, proposed only for the insensitive expediency of "getting things over with". Needless intervention subverts the importance of the role of family at the very onset of their lives together. There is no room for this kind of assembly-line mentality in the minds of most families who are seeking a gentle and normal birth for themselves and their babies.

HypnoBirthing preparation is beneficial for all families, including those who, because of genuine special circumstances, find themselves in the category of high-risk when their birthings take an unexpected turn. Should the course of birthing run differently from what was planned, and medical intervention or even surgical birth is required, HypnoBirthing enables parents to remain calm, relaxed and in control as they discuss options, evaluate the situation and make informed decisions concerning the birthing. The attitude of relaxed calm can help make the mother's recovery easier and reduce the necessity for medication throughout the recovery period.

The HypnoBirthing belief that birth should be looked upon as natural and healthy for the majority of women is expressed in the following Articles of Birth Affirmation.

ARTICLES OF BIRTH AFFIRMATION

- Birth is a natural, normal and healthy human experience.
  Women's bodies are created to conceive, nurture the
  development of babies, and to birth. Their bodies are not

flawed and destined to malfunction. In the absence of special circumstances, healthy women and their healthy babies deserve to be attended in a nurturing manner consistent with the status of their health.

- Families wishing to experience natural, unmedicated birth should be supported in their decision and encouraged through care and information to view birth as a positive, natural and even joyous experience. Their births should be allowed to naturally unfold in their own time, without undue chemical, chronological or emotional manipulation.

- Healthy women preparing for normal birth should be spared fear-provoking and intimidating discussions of abnormalities and dangers in the absence of any medical indication of such.

- Women, their partners and their babies are the principal players in this most significant experience. They deserve to be listened to and acknowledged as an integral part of the birthing care team.

- Pregnant couples should be encouraged to ask questions and express their wishes or concerns. They deserve to receive answers from their care providers that enhance their confidence and esteem as parents. Threats, sarcasm or other means of intimidation have no place in a nurturing caregiver/family relationship.

- Routine, non-evidence-based procedures, testing and drugs should be avoided during the pregnancies and birthings of healthy women unless there is specific, scientific indication for their use.

- Evidence shows that pre-born and newborn babies are aware, sensitive and feeling human beings who are participants in pregnancy and birth. Every effort should be made to accommodate the baby's need for physical and emotional safety and comfort, and to respect the importance of the family relationship.

- Care during birthing should be based solely on the well-being and needs of the mother and baby, and not upon time constraints or personal needs of caregivers or facility administration.

- Pregnant families need to be able to trust that information provided by their caregivers is truthful and dispensed only after full consideration of the particular woman's prognosis, the benefit-to-risk factor and the desire of the birthing family to birth naturally.

- Whenever circumstances allow, one or the other parent should participate in "receiving" their baby at birth if that is their wish.

- Women's bodies and, in particular, their vaginas, are as sacrosanct during pregnancy and birth as they are at any other time. Routine and unnecessary prodding and manipulation should be avoided in the absence of medical urgency.

- Families who are considered key players in their own birthings and who are afforded an opportunity to establish rapport, communication and a trusting relationship with their caregiver are least likely to leave their birthings in anger or with a feeling of betrayal, ready to explore litigation.

- It is a fundamental right of every family to expect that a care provider be willing to take the time to listen and hear, and, in response, to ask – yes, to ask – how they feel about particular medications, tests and procedures that involve the mother's health and safety, as well as that of her baby.

- Caregivers who are supportive of families wishing to have normal births deserve to be addressed in a spirit of mutual co-operation and trust. They have the right to know that should a true special circumstance occur, their advice and opinion will be respected and acted upon.

"What Eees All Dees Stuff?" The Power of Simplicity

> We are continuously amazed at the fact that our approach to our work is tremendously enhanced when we make thing simpler, not complicated.
>
> STEVE DYKSTRA

Several years ago, I met a woman in a breakfast room of a hotel outside of Seattle. As we talked, she asked why I was in Seattle. I told her that I was there to conduct a HypnoBirthing workshop at Bastyr University, and I asked why she was in Seattle. She told me that she was doing fund-raising for her mission in Africa.

My ears perked up, and I asked her to tell me about birthing in her village. She shrugged in a very cavalier way and asked, "What's there to tell? The women have their babies." I persisted. "How do they have their babies?"

In a rather matter-of-fact tone, she explained that a labouring mother goes about her usual daily routine until she feels the baby begin to move down. She then leaves what she is doing and finds a wall or support to lean her back against. Propped in this way, she extends her knees and crouches down, with her lower arms and elbows resting on the upper part of her slightly bent legs. As the baby emerges, she leans down with her extended hands and says, "Baby come". She receives her own baby.

I was excited to hear this because I honestly expected her to say that birth is as medicalised in her area as it is here in the States. I couldn't wait to get to Bastyr to tell my students. When I finished telling my story, one of the midwives in the class spoke up and said, "I have a story to go with that one, Mickey".

She told of once having a couple from Africa in her childbirth class. As she talked about the anatomy and physiology of labour and what happens at each stage, she could see that the husband was acting rather impatient. As she continued with details of complications and medications, the man began to roll his eyes and then tap his foot on the floor. His arms were tightly crossed on his chest. Everyone in the room was becoming aware of his apparent irritation, and the midwife felt that she had to address the situation. She asked him to share his thoughts.

The young man exploded, waving his arms into the air. "WHAT EES ALL DEES STUFF? IN AFRICA WE DOAN HAVE ALL DEES STUFF!! WE HAVE DE BABEE!!" And with that, he vigorously returned his arms to his chest, crossed them and emphatically thrust his head downward.

His message was simple. It goes to the heart of what we in HypnoBirthing frequently puzzle over: Why has all the "stuff" that denies the normalcy of birth and portrays it as an inevitably risky and dangerous medical event become a routine part of most childbirth education classes? Why are couples in a low- or no-risk category being prepared for circumstances that only rarely occur? Even more puzzling, why do parents accept the negative premise that birth is a dangerous, painful ordeal at best or a medical calamity at worst? Why do they blindly accept the "one-size-fits-all" approach?

If what couples are hearing in childbirth classes is far removed from what they want their birthing experiences to be, why do they spend so much time entertaining negative outcomes that can colour and shape their birth expectations and ultimately affect their birth experience? In other words, if it's not what they're wanting, why would they "go there"? In HypnoBirthing, we doan have all dees stuff, and deliberately so.

You will not find superfluous, fear-provoking "stuff" in HypnoBirthing. What is not there has been omitted intentionally; it is not an oversight. We believe the discussions that take place in many medical offices and hospital-based childbirth education programmes are the primary cause of much of the fear that parents bring to their birthings.

Discussions of possible hardships that almost never occur in a HypnoBirthing are not included in this book or in our outlines.

Lengthy explanations of difficult labours, described in harsh and confusing medical terms, have been left to other birthing programmes. Information of this kind creates a state of fear that all too often results in the anticipated complication – an unresponsive body and unrelenting discomfort. Presented in a medical environment, this information becomes a "prestige suggestion", meaning that it leaves an imprint that is more powerful than any other advice or stacks of printed literature to the contrary.

Many childbirth instructors feel pressured to act as information channels for their hospital and local physicians, so they teach a birth preparation class that is primarily designed to acquaint you with the "medical model". They educate you about the drugs, technological apparatus and medical procedures that are routinely used during conventional birthings at hospitals. In short, they teach you to be a good, acquiescing patient. In HypnoBirthing, we do not believe it is your responsibility to be a "good patient"; it is your responsibility to be a good *parent*.

In HypnoBirthing classes, you will discover a stress-free method of birthing that is devoted to helping you learn, through self-hypnosis and special Slow Breathing exercises, the art of "letting go" and opening yourself to the joy of experiencing birth calmly and serenely. Pain, described so thoroughly in other typical childbirth classes, does not need to be part of the universal birth story, and parents should not have to read, listen or take part in presentations that describe labour as intense and grueling.

HypnoBirthing helps you to frame a positive expectation and to prepare for birth by developing a trust and belief in your birthing body and in nature's undeniable orchestration of birthing. By teaching you the basic physiology of birth and explaining the adverse effect that fear has upon the chemical and physiological responses of your body, we help you to learn simple, self-conditioning techniques that will easily bring you into the optimal state of relaxation you will use during birthing. This will allow your birthing muscles to fully relax. In other words, we will help you prepare for the birth you plan and want for yourselves and your baby, rather than the birth that someone else directs. We will help you look forward to your pregnancy and birthing with joy and love, rather than fear and anxiety.

A DAD'S-EYE VIEW OF BIRTH

Conny's water released at 5:30 A.M., but nothing else was happening. She told me to go to work. At 9:00 A.M., she said she was having surges, but nothing regular. I decided to come home, just in case. We pulled stuff together for the hospital and decided to go to my parents' house, since they live only ten minutes from the hospital.

By the time we got to Dad's house, the surges had faded, and for the next few hours she didn't have even one. Conny was getting a little worried because in a few hours it would be twelve hours from the time her water released, and if things didn't start soon it could cause her to be induced at the hospital, which we didn't want.

After we ate, she lay down on the couch. We put on soft, instrumental music and started going through the relaxation scripts to put her at ease. Within ten minutes, she started having strong surges, five minutes apart. Within an hour, surges were about three to four minutes apart. By the time we reached the hospital, she was having surges every two minutes.

When she was assessed in the triage centre, Conny was already 7 to 8 centimetres open. She continued to do her slow balloon breathing through all of this, smiling and at ease in between the surges. It was unbelievable. It was just like we saw in the videos, but now it was so real.

We got into our delivery room at 6:00 P.M. The nurse set up the foetal monitor on her belly and then left us alone until Conny felt the need to start breathing the baby down. By 7:35 P.M., little Colin Emanuel Varga entered the world (only three and a half hours of labour) — no epidural, no episiotomy, no IV, no screaming baby, no pulling or pushing. He was seven pounds, three ounces and twenty inches long.

The doctor was absolutely fantastic. She was patient, understanding and encouraging, and used all the right terminology. Even the nursing staff was supportive. They were so surprised and impressed with this type of totally natural birth that we had a room full of nurses (between six to eight on a regular basis,

and most of those were just there to watch). Everything went so
well and so quick and so painless. As Conny put it: a lot of
pressure, but no pain.

HypnoBirthing really works. We had such a wonderful experience, and Colin is alert, content and happy. Best wishes to
the rest of you, and Happy HypnoBirthing.

MARK, CONNY and COLIN, CANADA

We receive a multitude of wonderful birth stories like the one
above almost daily. Their stories tell us that HypnoBirthing mums
do not experience labour in a typical way. The pattern is incon-
trovertible. HypnoBirthing mums are breaking every mould that
has been established by traditional birthing charts, scales and standards.

HypnoBirthings are often shorter, smoother and easier, and they
are experienced in peaceful relaxation that allows the mother's body
to function as nature intended. There is far less incidence of intervention because parents carefully choose care providers who support
their wishes for normal birth.

As a result of the aura of calm that our couples adopt, we are
seeing many confident, relaxed birthing women progress from
4 centimetres opened to 9 or 10 centimetres opened in a matter of
thirty minutes to an hour. We are also seeing mums who are ready
to start breathing their babies down to birth long before the
"appointed" 10 centimetres opened.

Even if, for some reason, a HypnoBirthing mum's labour is long
and slow, she remains comfortable, relaxed and energised throughout. The same is true of a short labour.

One of the nicest births – from the standpoint of relaxation and
comfort – that I have attended in a hospital setting lasted fifty-two
hours after the mother's membranes had released. The doctors were
willing to honour the couple's request for a normal birth, and the
mum allowed the baby to decide when to be born. After a reasonable amount of time had elapsed, the mum was put on antibiotics to
avoid the risk of infection. The family had almost two and a half
days of slow, lingering labour, but the birthing mother was totally

comfortable. Throughout their labour, this couple continued to use the methods of passing time that they had been taught in their classes.

On the shorter end of the time spectrum was a birth I attended that took more time for the administration of paperwork before and after the birth than it did for the birth. Again, this all took place while the mother was in complete calm and comfort. The confidence and relaxed attitude that this couple developed through their classes allowed them to simply and easily birth their baby in the midst of a bustling staff who insisted that the necessary paperwork be completed and that the mum not birth her baby until the doctor arrived. The baby had other plans and emerged exactly as he chose to, doctor or no doctor. In both of the above scenarios, the couples were totally happy with their birth experiences, and both babies made a calm, gentle entry into the world, free of intrusive interventions.

With such wonderful variations in the manner in which HypnoBirthing families experience labour and birth, we don't teach a first-time mum that she must plan on being in labour for at least twelve to twenty hours, if not more. Traditional birthing methods teach that a first stage of labour has, by itself, three distinct segments, slowly bringing a mother's body from 0 to 4 centimetres opened, then from 5 to 7 centimetres opened, and finally from 8 to 10 centimetres opened in a transition period. We don't teach numbers in HypnoBirthing. Experience with HypnoBirthing families shows that there are really no stages to labour. Labour stages are merely chartable milestones developed as assessment tools for medical care providers. For the mother, labour is one continuum, and when the birthing mother is deeply relaxed, birth unfolds. The thinning and opening phase simply spills into the birthing phase at whatever degree that the cervix is opened, and the mum breathes her baby down to crowning, sometimes with only a few unnoticeable birth breaths, to complete the baby's emergence.

Since you have chosen to birth normally, we will work with you in developing trust in your own intuitive birthing ability, talking of how you want to experience birthing, not about occurrences that rob you of your confidence and cast doubt on your ability to birth without fear.

Without all of *dees stuff,* you will come to understand the simple and true physiology of birth and, like other women who have freed themselves of the myths of birthing, you, too, will *have de babee,* smoothly, easily and in joy.

From Celebration to Fear:
A History of Women and Birthing

I include this brief account of the history of women and birthing, not to dwell on the negative past or to raise controversy, but rather as an explanation of how the societal influences of the early centuries caused birthing to go awry and left us clinging to a strong belief in the necessity of pain and anguish in childbirth.

Because the supposed "Curse of Eve" and its resulting impact upon birthing play such a major role in the minds of so many people in the Western world, it is important to examine this myth that has prevailed for so many centuries. In doing this, we learn that the belief in a curse that made pain a natural accompaniment of birthing has more to do with a certain time in history when religious men were trying to expand their dominance of society than it does in biology or observation.

Even today many people believe that to experience childbirth without pain would be contrary to the word and will of God. According to Helen Wessel, founder of Appletree Ministries and author of *The Joy of Natural Childbirth: Natural Childbirth and the Christian Family,* Hebrew scholars would differ. Wessel emphatically states, "There is no anthropological evidence to support the theological dogma that women of all cultures have universally regarded childbirth as an 'illness' or a 'curse'".

There is, in fact, much evidence to the contrary. In some of the less sophisticated societies where people have not been influenced by the beliefs of Western civilisation, for instance, women with bodies that are physiologically identical to those of Western women give birth with relatively no fanfare and with a minimum of discomfort.

To understand the events that led to our present beliefs surrounding the "sorrow" with which women have supposedly been cursed, we have to look back to as early as 3000 B.C., when women had their babies naturally and with a minimum of discomfort, unless there was complication. Wessel cites many references in the Bible that extol the blessing of motherhood, the procreation of life, and the affection between husband, wife and children. She points to the time of Moses, when Jewish women had their babies quite easily and within a relatively short period of time, often without assistance. Historical records of the period just prior to the time of Jesus indicate that births were often accomplished in less than three hours. There is no record of a "curse" having played any part in their beliefs or their birthings.

In other parts of the world – Spain, France, the British Isles and old Europe – the lives of the people centred on nature and motherhood. They honoured Mother Nature, Mother Earth and Mother Creator. Women were revered as the givers of life.

With no awareness of the link between intercourse and the conception of a child, it was believed that women brought forth children at will. As creators, they were thought to be connected to deity. Statues of the goddesses of these early people were of full-breasted women with bodies clearly depicting the ballooning abdomen of women about to give birth. These primal people regarded birthing as the highest manifestation of nature. When a woman gave birth, everyone gathered around her in the temple for the "celebration of life". Birthing was a religious rite, and not at all the painful ordeal it came to be years later.

Women were nurturers and healers, developing, brewing and administering medicine. All healing came by the hands and the healing spirit of women. They collaborated and exchanged learning, overseen by the "wise women" of the village. Men were the gatherers of food, herbs and building materials. Their roles were different, yet equal.

Even when men took the lead in early medicine, there was no change in the attitude toward birth. Neither Hippocrates nor Aristotle, leaders of the Grecian School of Medicine, wrote of pain in their notes on normal, uncomplicated birth. Are we to believe that the presence of pain in normal birthing simply escaped the notice of these learned men?

Hippocrates and Aristotle believed that the needs and the feelings of women in childbirth were to be accommodated. They advocated having support persons attend a labouring woman. In fact, Hippocrates was the first to organise and present formal instruction to women who engaged in midwifery. Aristotle wrote of the mind-body connection and emphasised the importance of deep relaxation during childbirth. In the event of complication, women were brought into a relaxed state so that the complication could be resolved and treated.

Within the last century before the birth of Jesus, another learned man from the Grecian School, Soranus, put the writings of Aristotle and Hippocrates into book form. Soranus stressed the importance of listening to the needs and feelings of women giving birth and advocated using the powers of the mind to achieve relaxation to bring about easy birthing. Like his predecessors, Soranus included no mention of pain, except when he wrote of abnormal or complicated birth. Women were treated kindly, gently and joyfully during the natural occasion of giving birth. This attitude prevailed for thousands of years.

At the end of the second century A.D., however, there arose a widespread wave of contempt against women, and particularly the midwives, healers and wise women who had been so instrumental to birth. The hatred, unfortunately led by some misguided early Christians, escalated into what would later become an actual holocaust of women where healers, who had previously held a very favourable position in society, were executed because of their caring and healing skills.

Literally, few stones were left unturned as the leaders set out to redefine the role of women in both religion and society. The stone temples and altars of the people who worshipped nature were destroyed, and the womanly icons were smashed and buried. To ascribe any importance to the laws or functions of nature became a serious offence, and all writings dealing with natural cures were seized and buried. Regrettably, Soranus's books met this sad fate, and the concept of natural birth was buried. It was at this time that St. Clement of Alexandria wrote: "Every woman should be filled with shame by the thought that she is a woman".

Law now demanded that women be segregated during pregnancy and isolated during birthing. With authority over all medical practice and healing firmly ensconced in the hands of the priests and monks, doctors had to obtain permission to administer to the "deserving ill".

Since women were labelled seductresses and the resulting pregnancy was seen as the product of "carnal sin", a labouring woman was not considered among the deserving ill. People in the medical field were forbidden to attend birthings, ensuring that no relief could be dispensed, even in the event of a complicated birth. Midwifery was abolished, leaving the labouring mother isolated, without support and terrified. By a series of decrees, birth, previously welcomed as a celebration of life, eroded into an excruciatingly painful, lonely and much-to-be-feared ordeal.

It was only at this time that what is now known as "The Curse of Eve" came to be embedded into biblical translations. Previously, there was no mention of a curse, except God's curse upon the ground and its implication that humankind would now have to work to survive. With the new translation, women were to pay the price of original sin, and it was, indeed, a high one.

Through his own study into the Bible and from his association with biblical scholars, Dick-Read learned that the Hebrew word *etzev*, used sixteen times in the King James I version, is translated to mean "labour, toil and work" throughout most Bibles, but when the same translators referred to childbirth, the word was interpreted to mean "pain, sorrow, anguish or pangs". Other scholars, too, point out that the prophets made no such reference to pain in their writings on childbirth. Wessel states that there was never an actual curse placed exclusively upon Eve. In Genesis, God uses the very same wording in speaking to Adam as to Eve. The translators, though, influenced by the terrible conditions surrounding birth, chose to translate the dictum delivered to Eve differently.

Finally, in the early sixteenth century, the lost writings of Soranus were discovered. The medical world took interest, and those in medicine who were driven by conscience defied the existing laws. The first book on obstetrics was written, based on the theories and teachings of the most profound medical philosophers and practitioners the world had yet known.

At this time, midwifery came back into practice, but it was looked upon as a dishonorable occupation "best suited to women to take care of the nasty business of giving birth". In Germany, where the largest number of executions of healers occurred, Martin Luther wrote, "If women become tired, or even die, it does not matter. Let them die in childbirth. That's what they are there for." He conceived a title for midwives that expressed the prevailing beliefs of the time and, in itself, suggested pain. *Weh mutters* was the name he attached to the women who attended birthing mothers. Literally translated from the German, *weh* means pain, and *mutter* means mother – "mothers of woe". There is no indication of the existence of this word prior to this time.

With the coming of the Renaissance and the "rebirth of learning", birthing women fared better, although even the advent of chloroform, widely used for all medical procedures, did nothing to relieve their plight. Chloroform was denied to women in labour. This attitude toward women and birthing was not limited to Europe. When it was suggested that pain relief be given to women in labour, a New England minister responded that to do so would rob God of the pleasure of their "deep, earnest cries for help". Once more, we see the misguided beliefs of man, not God, prevailing.

When we look back upon these events with our modern knowledge, we understand more clearly how fear of complication and resulting death, not fear of birthing, caused women to look upon labour with horror. Extreme fear created extreme tension, and the tension, in turn, resulted in a taut cervix, unable to perform its natural function. Those who lived through the ordeal, as well as those who witnessed it, attested to the agony that was experienced in birthing.

It wasn't until well into the middle of the eighteenth century that doctors were allowed to attend women, but most were reluctant. The stigma of male physicians being involved in obstetrics was strong. As a result, those doctors who found their way to obstetrics were usually inept or alcoholics, but it didn't matter because the conditions of birthing didn't matter. Birthing mothers were seen as insignificant in the world of medicine.

In the late 1800s, when Queen Victoria insisted that she be given chloroform when she birthed, the door opened for women to have anaesthesia in birthing. This, though, created another disaster that would last for years in European countries, as well as in the United States. Birthing began to move from the home into the hospital, not because birthing was too dangerous an experience to be accomplished in the home, but because the administration of anaesthesia made it too dangerous to be accomplished in the home. Inability to safely monitor the administration of anaesthesia led to all sorts of problems, including fatalities. So it was that women who sought anaesthesia had to leave their homes and go to hospitals. Husbands were no longer a part of the birthing scene, and families had little control over their own birthings. A new era and a new approach to the way in which birth would occur had its initiation.

Once in hospitals, birthing mothers met another unkind fate. Maternity wards in hospitals were appallingly dirty. Infections from something as simple as unwashed hands ran rampant. Many women who went to hospitals for safety and good medical treatment died from infection that came to be commonly called "childbed fever". The high rate of maternal and infant morbidity in hospitals was accepted because suffering and death in birthing were still believed to be decreed – in spite of the fact that there was a remarkably lower rate of complication or death among women who birthed in their own homes.

A 1913 study by the Carnegie Trust reported that while women and babies were dying in hospitals, birthing women in fishing villages and in the highlands of the British Isles, who had their babies in homes that they shared with lambs, chickens and other animals, experienced no deaths or major complications. Deaths in hospitals were the result of lack of sanitation and exposure to the contagion of illnesses of other patients, rather than complication or the danger of birthing. Nevertheless, deaths occurred, and the fear of death became even more strongly associated with giving birth.

It's impossible to even think that a woman at this time could approach the birthing experience with anything but the most terrifying fear, knowing that in the event of a complication, at best, she would experience outrageous suffering, and at worst, she may never live through the ordeal. It was clear that birthing was no longer considered a celebration of life. In the eyes of women themselves, a painful birthing was the sentence that women were to endure throughout eternity.

Much of the credit for changing birthing conditions belongs to a woman – Florence Nightingale. Nightingale re-established schools of midwifery and insisted that maternity wards adopt the same standards of sanitation and cleanliness as other wards in hospitals. Using her money-raising ability as clout, she saw to it that the inept, alcoholic doctors disappeared from the birthing scene and that women were treated kindly.

But it was too late. Once anaesthesia was generally available for birthing, the pendulum swung very quickly from lack of supervision to overprescription. Early administration of drugs and anaesthesia became the standard for all birthings – needed or not. Since it was believed that painful birthing was inevitable, women were given heavy doses of painkillers during the first part of labour and were administered general anaesthesia as soon as there was any indication of crowning. Drugged births, where babies were pulled from the birth path with instruments, became the rule. Relief for the labouring woman and expediency for the medical staff ruled the day and, to a large extent, still does.

Today, in spite of evidence to the contrary, an incredible number of people in maternal services, and even women themselves, continue to accept the myth that pain is an inevitable part of birthing. It is widely thought that the best a woman can do is depend upon care providers to help them get through the experience, rather than learn how to prevent adverse incidents beforehand.

Artificial inducement and augmentation are being routinely administered without evidence-based indication in far too many situations. These drugs introduce pain into the birthing and create a slippery slope whereby additional drugs may be necessary to quell the pain brought on by the first drug. As a result, many families come away from their birthing experience with stories tinged with apology, disappointment and rationalisation as to what "went wrong". They speak of long periods of terrible pain, the administration of multiple drugs, of uteruses that won't open, of surgical births, and mostly of feelings of helplessness. This kind of upheaval and, in some cases, trauma, cannot help but affect women and their babies.

Why are women having these experiences? Why do women's bodies, perfectly created to birth, shut down even before they start labour? Why do so many women require that their babies be extracted surgically – a procedure that forty years ago was so infrequent that it was regarded with surprise?

The answer can be found in one word: fear.

How we give birth matters! What our babies experience shapes who they are. What a mother experiences at the very transition from maiden to mother changes her. Gentle, natural birth unlocks something primal at our very core that makes mothering easier [and] makes families stronger. ... If parents would only realise that every single decision they make from conception onward influences the outcome of their birth, they could reclaim what they didn't even know was lost.

KIM WILDNER, MOTHER'S INTENTION

How Fear Affects Labour

To those who say it is just not possible to birth naturally and without pain, I say, "But what if we're right? Wouldn't it be wonderful"?

LORNE R. CAMPBELL, M.D.

Just today, I met with a vivacious young woman who is five months pregnant. She glowed as she talked about her pregnancy and how she has felt so wonderfully healthy. She spoke of all the things she is doing to prepare her body for birth – swimming, yoga, walking. In the middle of all of this happy conversation, she paused, clenched her fists and said, "But I can't even think about THAT day. I have totally blocked out all thought about the birth. I can't bear the thought of what it will be like. I am so scared."

"Terrified" is the more appropriate word to describe what women are feeling as they approach what should be among the most exciting moments of their lives. This young woman, obviously very sophisticated and very much in control of the events of her life, took on an air of helplessness when it came to the thought of birthing. Sadly, she represents women in many parts of the world. It is a travesty that manufactured fear, leading to manufactured consent, casts such a cloud over the otherwise joyful excitement that couples should feel as they anticipate becoming parents.

The belief in pain surrounding childbirth is so strong that, instead of questioning the validity of the concept, there have been many efforts to rationalise its importance and to attach some reason and higher purpose to it.

Some programmes teach methods that attempt to take your focus away from pain so that you will not be so aware of it. Others will tell you that pain is a very important signalling mechanism, a sort of biofeedback that alerts you to where you are in your labour. The theory is that if you can identify the degree of severity and the frequency of it, you will be better able to determine where you are in labour and what coping techniques you will employ to continue. Still others suggest that you look upon it as an unavoidable, but useful friend that can be tolerated, worked with and learned from. There are even those who revere pain in birthing and see it as a vehicle through which to achieve the empowerment of womanhood. It has been suggested that we learn to honour pain, as other societies do, for the strength it builds in our character. These programmes feel that because pain has to serve some purpose, it must be rationalised and accommodated in some way. For most women, these are not convincing arguments. Pain is still a four-letter word; accepting the belief that it is necessary creates the very situation they want to avoid.

For those who refuse to examine the theory that there is no physiological reason for pain in birthing, the way to accommodate it is to provide a plethora of drugs that the birthing mother can escape into. For the pregnant mothers looking forward to such relief, the drugs are offered, not as a last resort during labour, but rather as a menu, presented within the childbirth education class so that selections and decisions can be made early on. These mothers want to believe that the drugs won't cross the placenta and affect their babies. No one tells them that the placenta has no barrier. And so they go into their labours believing that their birthing bodies are inadequate, but they can be "delivered" by drugs and technology, even when these interventions take them further away from normal and gentle birth for their babies.

Occasionally one of the women in a HypnoBirthing class will ask, "Why don't we human beings have our babies the way cats and dogs and horses and other animals do? There's nothing wrong with their labours." My reply is always the same: "Yes, why don't we?"

Medical professionals have long stood by the argument that pain is considered the "watchdog of medicine". Pain, they tell us, sends a signal that something is wrong. If that is true, we must make an exception for all other mammals for which labour is a natural, normal function. We know that horses and other "dumb" animals will delay the start of their labours or shut them down when they

The Uterine Layers

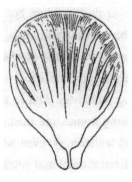

The outer longitudinal muscle fibres

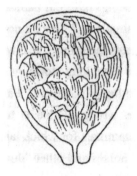

The middle muscle layers, interwoven with blood vessels

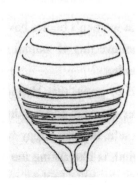

The inner circular muscle layers found mostly at the lower part of the uterus

don't feel comfortable with their environment or they feel endangered. Is it not unreasonable to think that women's bodies have that same instinctual capacity? Why do we believe this of animal mothers, yet refuse to consider it for human mothers?

I am frequently asked to prove that HypnoBirthing works – that eliminating fear and other stressors and building trust in the birthing process results in a truly safe, healthy, happy-baby and happy-mother outcome. This, in my mind, is like asking me to take a finely tuned, precision instrument that has been broken and prove that it would work perfectly had it not been broken in the first place.

Birth has been broken. The spirit of women with respect to their innate birthing power has been broken. We can do nothing about the millions of broken births that have already taken place, but by seriously looking at the effect of fear – the powerful emotion that clouds our thinking and causes the birthing body to break down and deviate from its natural course – perhaps we can keep the finely tuned, precision bodies of women whole for future generations.

YOUR MARVELLOUS BIRTHING DEVICE: THE UTERUS

Your uterus is perfectly designed to assist you to birth your baby. When we understand the way in which the uterus functions naturally when unencumbered by fear, the concept of easier, more comfortable childbirth immediately becomes obvious, and, therefore, attainable. *This very brief explanation and the facing illustrations are, indeed, the crux of our entire programme.* It is exactly this process of your body that you will work with during labour. This is the way the birthing muscles are designed to work – in perfect harmony.

There are three layers of muscle in the uterus. The two layers with which we will be concerned are the outer layer, with muscles that are vertical (aligned up and down with your baby), and the inner layer, with muscles that are horizontally circular (surrounding the baby).

The circular muscles of the inner layer are found in the lower portion of the uterus. As the illustrations show, the circular muscles are thickest just above the opening, or neck, of the uterus, called the cervix. In order for the outlet of the uterus to open and permit the baby to easily move down, through and out of the uterus into the birth path, these lower, thicker muscles have to relax and thin.

The stronger muscles of the outer layer of the uterus are vertical fibres, with a stronger concentration at the top. They go up the back and over the top of the uterus. As these muscles tighten and draw up the relaxed circular muscles at the neck of the uterus, they cause the edges of the cervix to progressively thin and open. In an almost wavelike motion, the long muscle bands shorten and flex to nudge the baby down, through and ultimately out of the uterus. It is this tightening motion that many HypnoBirthing mothers report as being the only sensation that they experience during the thinning and opening phase of labour.

When the labouring mother is in a comfortable state of relaxation, the two sets of muscles work in harmony, as they were intended. The surge of the vertical muscles draws up, flexes and expels; the circular muscles relax and draw back to allow this to happen. The cervix thins and opens. Birthing occurs smoothly and easily.

The Slow Breathing technique that you will learn and practise in your classes is designed to help you to work in concert with these birthing muscles. Combined with the relaxation practise you will do on a daily basis at home, this will help you learn to bring your body into a relaxed state that can make your surges more effective and substantially shorten your labour. You will learn to visualise the lower circular muscles as soft, blue satin ribbons, flexible and totally non-resistant to the draw of the upper muscles.

FEAR: THE ENEMY OF THE BIRTHING ROOM

We have seen how the birthing muscles are beautifully orchestrated to work. Now let's look at what happens when the birthing mum is tense and fearful.

The effect of fear upon labour is not subtle, insidious or complex. We see it in front of us with every labour that is delayed in starting or that later slows or stalls. Yet this obvious emotion, one of the strongest and most debilitating that we know, is basically ignored. Instead of being helped to recognise the harmful effects of fear upon the body, mothers are asked to surrender themselves to drugs, technology and manipulation to force their bodies to do what they are naturally capable of doing when left to their own means and when the circumstances are "right" for birthing.

The negative physical effect of fear on labour can be traced to the function of the body's Autonomic Nervous System (ANS). The ANS is the communication network within our bodies. Its main function is to interpret messages it receives, determine what action should be taken as a result of the message, and then immediately communicate that directive to the other systems of the body. The responses to impulses that are transmitted through the ANS are not subject to our conscious control and are, therefore, involuntary.

For the purpose of looking at the impact of stress upon birthing, as well as the beneficial effect of calm, we'll need to look at the two subsidiary systems within the ANS – the Sympathetic system and the Parasympathetic system. These systems control those responses that cause us to accelerate or slow our breathing, to blink our eyes, to step up or reduce our heartbeat, to arrest or maintain our digestive processes, and to carry out many other functions of the body.

The Sympathetic system is triggered when we are stressed, frightened or startled. Therefore, I call this part of the system the "Emergency Room". It is the role of the Sympathetic system to act as the body's defence mechanism. It instantly creates the "fight, flight or freeze" response within the body. When it is in motion, it causes the pupils in the eye to dilate, increases the speed and the force of the heart rate, and causes the body to startle and move defensively. It suspends activities such as digestion. Most important, it closes arteries going to organs that are not essential for defence. It prepares the body to deal with emergencies and danger. It is designed to save your life.

The activities of the Emergency Room put you into a state of alert. For that reason, you should be spending no more than 2 to 5 per cent of your life in the Emergency Room. It is like a "rainy day fund", and it shouldn't be tapped into on a regular basis.

On the other hand, the Parasympathetic system, which I call the "Healing Room", keeps the body and mind in a state of harmony and balance. It maintains the body functioning in a state of calm, slowing the heart rate, reducing stimulation, slowing the firing of harmful neuropeptides, and, in general, keeping us in a state of well-being. The Healing Room restores and maintains the normal

The Automatic Nervous System consists of two parts

Parasympathetic   Sympathetic

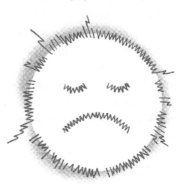

The Healing Room   The Emergency Room
95% to 98%   2% to 5%

functions of our bodies. We should be living 95 to 98 per cent of our lives in the Healing Room.

How does this relate to birthing? The Sympathetic part of the nervous system responds, not just to actual threats, but to *perceived* threats. In other words, the negative messages that a mother constantly receives are processed as being real. Over time, these negative messages become part of her belief system and compromise her body's chemical balance on a regular basis. They affect her emotional state and that of her pre-born baby.

When the mother approaches labour with unresolved fear and stress, her body is already on the defensive, and the stressor hormone, catecholamine, is triggered. Her body is sent into the "fight, flight or freeze" response. It is believed that catecholamine is secreted in large amounts prior to and during labour.

When circumstances are such that neither "fight" nor "flight" are appropriate, as in the case of labour, the body naturally chooses the third option: "freeze". Since the uterus has never been designated as part of the defence mechanism of the body, blood is directed away from it to the parts of the body involved in defence. This causes the arteries going to the uterus to tense and constrict, restricting the flow of blood and oxygen. Labour and birthing nurses and midwives have told me of seeing uteruses of frightened birthing women that are white from lack of blood, just as a person who is experiencing extreme fright often has the blood drain from his face.

With limited oxygen and blood, vital to the functioning of the muscles in the uterus, the lower circular fibres at the neck of the uterus tighten and constrict, instead of relaxing and opening as they should. The upper vertical muscles continue to attempt to draw the circular muscles up and back, but the lower muscles are resistant. The cervix remains taut and closed.

When these two sets of muscles work against each other, it causes considerable pain for the labouring mother. The situation can also have an adverse effect on the baby. The upper muscles push to expel, forcing the baby's head against the tightly closed lower muscles that refuse to budge. In addition to the pain that this causes for both mother and baby, labour can be drawn out, or it can even shut down. Thus, we hear from mothers whose labours end in a surgical birth lament, "My uterus wouldn't open". Limited oxygen in the uterus also means that the supply of oxygen to the baby is compromised. Over a period of time, this can be a cause for concern. The situation often is labelled "failure to progress" (FTP), and it usually results in intervention. It is interesting to note that the very same initials, FTP, are used to abbreviate both Grantly Dick-Read's Fear–Tension–Pain Syndrome and the failure to progress that it causes. What labour needs is not more urgency or prompting to "move things along", but more awareness of the importance of calm, relaxation, gentle encouragement and assurance that actually can move the labour along faster.

Regrettably, Dick-Read did not live long enough to see his theory buttressed with the discovery of endorphins. Still more regrettable is that, even with this knowledge in hand today, few medical caregivers are opening their minds to the relationship that exists between the birthing experience and the ANS, with its ability to secrete endorphins, the "feel-good" hormones that relax the muscles and allow the body to open, as well as the stressor hormone catecholamine.

Attempts to speed the birth of a baby only result in more pain for the mother and the baby, and frustration on the part of caregivers, as the baby's head pushes against muscles not yet relaxed and open enough to accommodate it. HypnoBirthing allows for the body to work at its own pace and facilitates easier birthing by using relaxation and visualisation to speed the release of endorphins and effect an even shorter labour.

You and your birthing companion will be taught how to identify emotional stress before and during labour and how to release it. You will learn how to bring yourself into a deepened relaxation. When you are free of fear, you can achieve a relaxed state from the very onset of labour. Verbal and physical cues that you and your partner have practised will help you to maintain a state of calm from the very start, as constricting hormones are overridden by your body's natural relaxants.

Learning to understand the benefits of living in the Healing Room – and avoiding people and situations that place you in the Emergency Room – is a skill that will infuse calm into your everyday life. It will greatly enhance your relationship as a family, as well as ensure a calm and gentle birth.

Releasing Fear

If a mother fights with others while she is pregnant, the
baby will come out fighting in childbirth, causing much
pain. The baby will grow up fighting and arguing.

ROGU, AS QUOTED IN MAMATOTO

Preparing women for birthing by educating them in the true physiology of labour was the backbone of Dick-Read's work. For many
women who were preparing for natural birthing in the 1950s, that
appeal to their intellect was enough to make them break with traditional attitudes and bring their children into the world
unmedicated and alert. It was simpler then. Most babies came into
the world with the assistance of the family doctor, a person who was
probably known to the birthing mother since she, herself, was a
child. While women did not expect that birth would be a picnic,
they were not terrified of the experience, and families of three or
four children were not uncommon. Free of debilitating fear, they
often were able to bring their babies to crowning with little fuss, and
were anaesthetised only in time for the doctor to arrive and extract
the baby with forceps. Those who subscribed to the philosophy of
natural birth were free of fear, free of anaesthesia and, for the most
part, free of the discomfort of labour.

If you are like most pregnant women, you will find that as you
move through these days and months of pregnancy, you will be
met with a whole new set of feelings, anxieties, doubts, questions,
decisions and tasks that you never had to consider before. Some of
these will centre on your pregnancy, labour and birthing, but there
may be more that will cause you to look at the many transforma-
tional experiences that bringing a baby into your life will present.

This is natural. As you prepare your mind and body for your baby's birth, you will want to be ready in this regard also – free of any fears, reservations or limiting thoughts.

It's helpful for both you and your partner to be able to identify feelings, experiences or recollections that may be painful or hurtful, thus limiting your ability to approach birthing free of harmful emotions. Take a look at those emotions that may foster a feeling of uneasiness, meet them head-on and release any conflict you may be harbouring (consciously or subconsciously) because of them. Once you have been able to work through and resolve lingering emotions, limiting thoughts, experiences or memories that could stand in the way of an easy birthing, you will have a better sense of your own ability to approach the birth of your baby with trust and confidence.

Thoroughly search your inner feelings to discover the areas that you feel very confident about and those that you need to work through so that you can resolve any fears or misgivings that you are holding. Brushing aside matters that concern you may help you to get through your pregnancy, but these concerns can easily surface as fears when you are in labour, and they can affect the course of your labour. You will want to take advantage of the opportunity to talk with your partner, your birthing companion or a good friend who can help you explore and discuss any thoughts that could be troubling you.

Your HypnoBirthing practitioner will help you inventory and identify those areas of your life that could possibly serve as obstacles. The practitioner will help you work with fear-release sessions in class. If you still feel you need some assistance in releasing lingering fears after you do the sessions in class and talk with your partner and friends, ask your practitioner for a private session. If you are not able to work with a trained practitioner, you may find it helpful to seek the counsel of a hypnotherapist to do release work with you. A fear-release hypnotherapy session is truly one of the most effective ways of eliminating toxic emotions.

Listed below are just a few areas of concern to pregnant women that surfaced in the early nineties as a result of Dr. Louis Mehl-Madronna's study on turning breech babies with hypnosis. Your own inventory may reveal other issues that you would like to resolve.

- **Your own birth** – What stories have you heard about your own birth? Are they positive and encouraging, or negative and frightening? Do you feel that you will duplicate your mother's labour? If what you've been told is less than encouraging, you might want to work on establishing that you are *not* your mother, and this is not *her* pregnancy. You are an entirely different person at a different time and under different circumstances.

- **Others' birth stories** – Have you been surrounded with stories of joyful birthing, or have family members impressed upon you "family patterns" of long labours, back labour, severe pain and medical intervention? Again, you do not need to assume the experiences of the people who are relating these stories. There is no reason to believe that you will birth as they did. Work at checking those kinds of thoughts so that you don't bring their past baggage into your birthing.

- **Previous labours** – Has your own experience with labour been easy and satisfying, or are you carrying recollections of an arduous ordeal? If you had a less than satisfying labour, take hope in the fact that you are better prepared for an easier birth this time, and you now can approach birthing with more knowledge and planning than you did before. Make your HypnoBirthing skills work for you, and get rid of the memories of the previous birth or births.

- **Parenting** – Did you learn positive attitudes toward parenting that you feel comfortable with? If not, do you feel less than adequate about your ability to be a good parent? Do you feel overwhelmed? Quite often people who did not grow up with good role models can learn a great deal from less-than-great models about what they wouldn't want to do in their own parenting. Turn it into a positive factor.

- **Support** – Do you feel secure with the support that your partner and/or family will provide? Is there someone who will share the responsibilities of caring for the baby? Sometimes just tackling the issue and letting people know you will want and need support will resolve the matter. In other circumstances, take advantage of the opportunity to see what strengths you must build to effectively provide your own best support.

- **Marriage/relationship** – Is your marriage/relationship secure, loving and mutually nurturing? Are you confident that your relationship is strong and that it will weather the additional concerns of raising a child? Are there some agreements you need to work out? Have you really "talked"? Perhaps a confidence-building session can help you sort out your abilities. Working together in HypnoBirthing can bring about a stronger bond than you ever believed could exist.

- **Career** – Will you be able to continue to pursue your own goals with reorganising and planning? Will your plans need to be put on hold? Are you ambivalent about going back to work or staying home with your baby? Sorting through these questions can help you reconcile with what you really feel you want to do.

- **Housing** – Is there room in your home, as well as in your heart, for your new baby? Can accommodations be easily made? Can you make changes? If not, express those wishes and you'll soon see how your circumstances can change.

- **Medical care** – Do you feel comfortable with your present medical care provider? Do you feel that he or she is supportive of your plans for your birthing? Are there lingering doubts? Have you discussed your preferences for a natural birth with this person and made your wishes known? Are your decisions fear-based or confidence-based?

- **Finances** – Do you see finances being "stretched" as a result of adding another person into your life? Ask your HypnoBirthing practitioner about some abundance work. The Law of Attraction can help in this regard: Remember, you get what you say and see.

- **Prior relationships** – Are you carrying around some unhappy memories of an earlier relationship or an experience that has left hurtful thoughts? It's time to eliminate those thoughts and let them go through a release session.

- **Personal experience of abuse** – Are you harbouring unhappy memories of an experience of physical or sexual abuse? Because these experiences are so associated with your body, bitter or hurtful memories can easily rise to the surface during birthing. Birthing is one of the most profoundly physical experiences you will know in your lifetime. Overwhelming feelings of helplessness, inadequacy and fear have the ability to make your body shut down or resist. It is important that you do release work with a qualified hypnotherapist before you advance any further into your pregnancy.

Please take this assessment seriously. Your mind and body work best when both are in harmony so that you can approach your birthing as free of limiting thoughts and emotions as possible.

The Power of the Mind

The mind is capable of anything – because everything is in
it, all the past, as well as all the future.

JOSEPH CONRAD

We've just seen the power of the mind, specifically how fear can
interrupt the body and the natural birth process. The good news is
that the opposite is also true: Positive thought and relaxation can help
the body and enhance its ability to birth freely, effectively and with
no ill effects. That is, after all, what HypnoBirthing is all about.

As far back as early Grecian times, relaxation, visualization and
quiet recitations have been used by priests to aid people in ridding
themselves of illnesses. Tribal Indian customs and "old wives'" super-
stitions were used for centuries to bring about physical and
emotional healing. Now, many years later, we are coming to an
awareness and acceptance of the ways in which self-hypnosis can
physiologically affect tissues and mentally reprogramme behaviours
that are impeding our success. Dr. Bruce Lipton, a well-known
author, is in the forefront today with his work on the effect of the
mind in changing tissues at the cellular level.

Researchers are discovering, through studies of everything from
memory to dreams to subtle eye movements, that the mind and the
images held within it can largely determine your success or failure in
life. Motivational consultants, Olympic coaches and other sports
trainers, as well as people in medicine, are realising that visualisation – the process of mentally producing pictures of a desired goal
or result – is an important factor in the achievement of that goal,
and they are routinely incorporating self-hypnosis and visualisation
sessions into their programmes.

Educational psychologists have conducted visualization studies suggesting that extrapolative learning – the method of mentally working through a physical process – can produce a response within muscles that is similar to what would occur if the routine were physically practised.

During self-hypnosis, the brain and nervous system are saturated with a picture of a specific, ideal sensory vision that seems so real, it becomes imprinted in the brain. This occurs exactly the way that real experiences become embedded within the memory of the sub-conscious. When a person is in a relaxed state, the mind more easily adapts to the imagery and accepts the suggested vision as being real. The assimilation of the repeated image causes the belief in the desired outcome.

Though neuroscientists are just beginning to understand how this occurs on a cellular level, sufficient study of this phenomenon has resulted in a very clearly defined set of Laws of the Mind. The concept of easier birthing through the positive application of these Laws is changing the view of birthing and is the basis of HypnoBirthing.

THE POWERFUL LAWS OF THE MIND

The application of four specific Laws of the Mind has a direct effect on changing the view of birthing, and these Laws are the basis for much of the work that we do in HypnoBirthing.

The Law of Psycho-Physical Response
The Law of Harmonious Attraction
The Law of Repetition
The Law of Motivation

THE BODY FOLLOWS THE MIND: THE LAW OF PSYCHO-PHYSICAL RESPONSE

The process of achieving desired results through application of the Laws of the Mind can be more clearly understood by examining the Robot Theory forwarded by Dr. Al Krazner in his book, *The Wizard Within*. The Robot Theory is based on the Law of Psycho-Physical

Response. This law states that for every suggestion, thought or emotion one entertains, there is a corresponding physiological and chemical response within the body. This is the most important Law of the Mind in regards to birthing.

The body is the action component of the mind. What is experienced in the body is determined in the mind. Therefore, what the mind chooses to accept or perceive as being real, the robot body, accordingly, responds to. The mind does not have the ability to act. Therefore, it sends messages to the body demanding action. The body, in turn, plays out the thought. Pavlov's experiment with the dogs that eventually became conditioned to salivate in anticipation of receiving food at the ringing of a bell is perhaps the most commonly recognized example of this mind-body connection.

We experience this law almost every day of our lives. I'm sure it would not be difficult for you to recall any number of incidents when a loud, sudden noise or the unexpected appearance of a person or an object in your path caused you to startle, duck, draw back or involuntarily cry out.

A dad in one of my classes described experiencing an instant and noticeable physical response when seeing the flashing lights of a police car in his rearview mirror at a time when he was driving well beyond the speed limit. It was not until he pulled over to the side of the road and the policeman continued past him that he became aware of how strong a physiological effect his thoughts had created within his body. He could feel the accelerated pounding of his heart, the dampness accruing at his underarms, the white-knuckle grip he had on the steering wheel, and the long, continuous intake of breath, without exhaling. He was also hugely aware of the relief he felt as he exhaled and his shoulders receded back into the frame of his body. When the mind no longer perceived that he was being threatened, he relaxed back into a state of calm.

Of course, the most obvious example of the psycho-physical response is the one that has brought you to HypnoBirthing class to prepare for your baby's birth – sexual arousal. When the mind entertains a sexual thought and a subsequent visualization, the body responds by preparing for the sex act with the male experiencing penile erection and the female experiencing lubrication of the vaginal wall. This all comes naturally, with the robot body acting out the desires of the mind. It is part of the master plan for all reproduction.

Utilising this Law of the Mind so that it works with you and for you, and not against you, during your birthing is essential. If the mind is dwelling on fearful, negative images of birth, the body is thrown unintentionally into a defence mode. The physical response then becomes the antithesis to normal birthing – tension.

You will become skilled in using your own natural abilities to bring your mind and body into psycho-physical harmony so that the thoughts you use in practise are those that will condition your body and your mind to create endorphins – those neuropeptides that create a feeling of well-being. You will learn special deepening techniques that will help you to connect with your baby and work with your body to bring yourself even deeper as your labour advances.

THE POWER OF LANGUAGE: THE LAW OF HARMONIOUS ATTRACTION AND THE LAW OF REPETITION

Words and thoughts are powerful and profoundly affect our every-day experiences and beliefs. Equally significant is the harm that is created by the negative energy of the confusing, harsh and fright-ening words of conventional birthing.

A second Law of the Mind, the Law of Harmonious Attraction, is very much in evidence here. This law states that what we put out in the way of thinking and speaking creates energy that comes back to us in the same form in subsequent experiences. This is what I call the "echo effect" or the "boomerang effect". Whatever thought or emotion you throw out to the world will come back to you exactly as you first proposed it. Applying this law on a daily basis is impor-tant. The best advice, according to Esther Hicks in the *Abraham-Hicks Material*, is, "If it's not what you're wanting, don't go there".

Words have energy, power and vibrations that translate into action. Regardless of whether you are the person speaking or the person being spoken to, the sound and vibration of what is being said cause an emotional response within your mind, and a physio-logical and chemical response within your mind-body. Over time, the frequency of that response becomes part of your belief system, strengthening itself each time a similar vibration is accepted. It then attracts more of the same.

Even when we silently engage in self-talk, our words have force. Each time we speak to ourselves in a less-than-complimentary way – "Are you stupid, or what"?– or use similar self-denigrating words, we leave an imprint of inadequacy upon our subconscious.

You can see this demonstrated as you listen to the people around you. Notice that healthy people rarely speak of becoming ill. However, people who are not healthy frequently punctuate their conversation with talk of their physical ailments. Think about the phrase, "The rich get richer, and the poor get poorer". Rich people don't often speak of being poor or not being able to afford goods. On the other hand, poor people, or people who "think poor", regularly end thoughts of spending with the phrase, "I can't afford it". They remain in that situation and go through life affording very little. It is therefore essential that you keep your thoughts and language focused on what you do want rather than creating wasted, negative energy around circumstances that you don't want.

The little ditty that you may have heard on the playground when you were a child – "Sticks and stones may break my bones, but names will never hurt me" – may be a good comeback as temporary defence against words that sting, but, physiologically, it is not true. Caustic, belittling, frightening and abusive words do, indeed, hurt and can cause a lasting imprint. Tell a baby just learning to walk or beginning to accomplish tasks on his own that he is clumsy or a klutz, and after a while, the child begins to feel clumsy and moves in ways that are clumsy. Tell him that his everyday, normal bodily functions are "smelly and disgusting", and he begins to feel bad about his body and himself for having created a disgusting situation. The negative imprint takes hold, stays with him and grows. The more potent the thought, the more potent the imprint.

Concepts that you are exposed to repeatedly in many places and from many sources become part of a conditioning that becomes embedded in your thoughts over time. The Law of Repetition governs that process. It is important for you to recognise that frequency does not necessarily equal fact.

The association of pain with childbirth is an example of a universally held conditioning, and it has become the source of needless

suffering because of the myths that have grown up around it. By the
same token, if you listen to affirmations of positive, gentle birth on
a daily basis, it will contribute to positive conditioning.

Words and suggestions set off a chain of feelings, beliefs and
reactions that can be uplifting, encouraging and supportive – or
totally debilitating. The following chart shows the flow of energy
and the effect of words.

Words create thoughts and emotions; repeatedly entertaining the
same thoughts conjures up feelings. Over time, these feelings
become beliefs. We begin to act out those beliefs by our behaviour.
Our behaviour shapes our experiences. Positive behaviour creates
positive experiences; negative behaviour creates negative experiences. Hence, in HypnoBirthing, we focus only on the positive.

For all of these reasons, HypnoBirthing parents learn to use language that more nearly describes what is happening within the
birthing mother's body during birth. This gentle language is more
meaningful to parents than language that is couched in medical
academicism – appropriate for the medical caregivers in communicating with each other, but frightening and potentially harmful to
the birthing family.

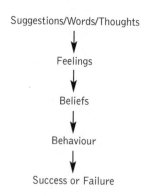

Suggestions/Words/Thoughts

↓

Feelings

↓

Beliefs

↓

Behaviour

↓

Success or Failure

The language you use and the language you hear from people
around you, including caregivers and childbirth educators, keep
your mind in a state of calm, or, conversely, trigger a state of unrest,
stress and fear. Learn to choose your words carefully and associate
with people who reinforce your own positive thinking about
birthing. If you are being bombarded by people who want to tell
you birth horror stories, suggest that you wait until after you have

your baby to exchange birth stories. Don't get pulled into those kinds of conversations.

This kind of thinking, speaking and living, as well as the support that you give to each other, will help you to work together toward a positive birth experience. This calmness will be there for you during birthing, and it spills over into every aspect of your family life.

To truly embrace the concept of gentle, normal birth, learn to think and speak in the kinder, softer word substitutes that appear on the list that follows. As you become accustomed to this language, you will become aware of the importance of this mental transition.

MEDICALISED LANGUAGE	HYPNOBIRTHING LANGUAGE
Instead of:	**Use:**
Contraction	Uterine Surge or Wave
Coach	Birth Companion
Catch the Baby	Receive the Baby
Deliver/Delivery	Birth/Birthing
Due Date	Birthing Time/Month
Pain or Contractions	Pressure/Sensation/Tightening
Water Breaking/Rupturing	Membranes Releasing
Birth Canal	Birth Path
Pushing	Birth Breathing
Complications	Special Circumstances
Mucous Plug	Uterine Seal
Bloody Show	Birth Show
Transition	Near Completion/Nearly Complete
Effacing/Dilating	Thinning/Opening
Foetus	Pre-born/Unborn Baby
Primip/Multip	First-/Second-Time Mum
Clients/Patients	Parents
Braxton-Hicks	Pre-Labour Warm-Ups
Kegels	Pelvic Floor Exercises
Neonate	Newborn
False Labour	Practice Labour

Birth-savvy mothers who value totally unmedicated and intervention-free birthing have a new term for it – "Pure Birth".

WHAT YOU WANT IS WHAT YOU GET: THE LAW OF MOTIVATION

The Law of Motivation also affects the physical body's capabilities. We have all read accounts of nearly impossible feats accomplished by people who risked their own lives to save the life of a child. When the mind is highly motivated, the body responds properly.

Consider the football player who sprains an ankle at the beginning of the last quarter of the game. Because his conscious attention and motivation is totally focused on playing the game and winning, he may feel the pressure of the swelling of the ankle but feels no pain. His mind has narrowed its focus and is accepting only the suggestion that he must remain in the game and play his hardest. His ankle does not accept the sharp twist as a source of pain because only the mind is able to think or react to pain stimuli. If there is no pain stimuli, he feels no pain. It is not until the game is over and the motivation to put all of his energy into winning the game is no longer necessary that his mind is redirected, the message of the sprain is relayed to the mind, the mind interprets it, and sends it back, and he begins to feel the discomfort.

When we examine motivation to see how it affects the way in which a woman births, we need only to look at a story that received national news coverage a few years ago. It involved a very pregnant young woman who was attending a prom when she went into labour. She excused herself, left the dance floor and went into the ladies' room where she proceeded to have her baby, quickly, quietly and unbeknownst to anyone else. Her fear of being detected created a motivation far stronger than any fear she may have had of the birthing itself. And so her baby was born easily and in very little time. She was able to accomplish the birth and return to the prom activities after only a brief period of labour. Her mind never accepted, or even considered, that there would be any impediments to this birth or that she would experience the long, typical labour that our society has come to expect, especially for a woman having a first baby.

While it is difficult to believe, we sometimes see the reverse of the previous example. If motivation is accompanied by a "secondary benefit", a person can actually bring about what, for most people, would be an unwanted situation – an illness, a bad outcome, a hardship. Without consciously being aware of it, "victims" of the secondary benefit can create circumstances that allow them to accomplish what they consider is a better end, even though it means they endure less than optimal circumstances.

I once worked with a woman who was referred to my office by a specialist from a leading eye clinic. She was diagnosed with hysterical blindness. The woman had been seen by several eye specialists throughout New England, and not one of them could find a pathological reason for her inability to see. During her first office visit, while in hypnosis, she revealed that she had been living in loneliness for years because her children were all too busy with their own lives to visit her. She was disappointed in not being able to *see* her children and her grandchildren. When she became blind, all of that changed. Her family visited regularly, and even her son who lived in the same town but was the most infrequent visitor, dropped in almost every day. Through several hypnosis sessions she was able to realise that her blindness was causing her a tremendous hardship that she no longer needed. She gradually regained her vision, continued to enjoy visits with her family and began to function as a normally sighted, happy person.

Could this kind of situation occur during pregnancy and birthing? It definitely can and occasionally does. If a pregnant woman wants and needs to be pampered, "waited upon" and coddled, and buys into the concept that pregnancy is an abnormal condition and she is "ill", the attention that she gains during a troublesome pregnancy and a difficult birthing can definitely make it all worthwhile in her mind. She barely tolerates her pregnancy and constantly proclaims her annoyance at all the aches, pains and other pregnancy "disorders", while she uses body language that demonstrates her plight. Family members often contribute to this scenario by cautioning the woman that she must "give in" to her frailty during this precarious time of her life.

Several years ago, a mum came to my classes talking about the horrendously long and difficult births her mother and all of the women in her family experienced. This was the centrepiece of her conversation week after week. As I got to know her family, I saw that all the women in the family talked in "victim" language. In spite of the fact that their birth stories were horrific, they were delighted to tell all of the details, each one surpassing the other, and each rushing in to grab her opportunity to tell how bad her pregnancies and birthings were. The mum and dad appeared to embrace the HypnoBirthing philosophy, but I was not surprised that her birthing story was one that could easily match and top those of her family members. The drama surrounding the birth was incredible, and there was a gathering of family and friends invited in to observe the performance. It was more important for this young woman to be able to remain in good standing in the sorority of her family and friends than it was to remain outside the group and to birth her baby calmly and peacefully as she had prepared.

This is not to say that all labours that are drawn out and difficult have behind them some secondary benefit. Nevertheless, it is important to assess your own motivation and intent as you approach your birthing and consider, in light of all we've spoken of here, how you will apply these Laws of the Mind so that they work for you.

Motivation is closely tied to your intent and your self-image. It is said that a woman births pretty much the same way that she lives life. For that reason, it is imperative that you take the time to do an assessment of how you see yourself and whether this image is productive for you or counterproductive. Much of the determining aspects of how you will make important choices concerning your birthing are factored on how you regard birth and your own role in this experience.

Two models – the whole-person model and the dependent model – determine how you will approach your pregnancy and birthing. Review each model and evaluate which traits you want to strengthen and expand upon as you make important decisions regarding your baby and your birthing. The model you choose to follow will be invaluable to you as you continue your adventure into pregnancy, birthing and lifelong parenting.

Dependent Model	Whole-Person Model
uninformed and unknowing	knowledgeable
submissive	powerful
passive onlooker	involved
conforming	forward thinking
reconciled	fulfilled
easily led	directing
vulnerable	trusting
helpless	self-sufficient
vacillating	decisive
threatened	confident
embarrassed	assertive
resigned	satisfied

SOME NOTES ON SELF-HYPNOSIS

There is a great deal of misconception about self-hypnosis. This is because the only exposure that many people have had to hypnosis, in general, is what they've seen as entertainment – stage hypnosis. Without going into detail, I will simply remind you that the people who are on the stage during a stage show are volunteers, there to have a good time. Since all hypnosis is self-hypnosis, it is easy for them to accept the roles that the hypnotist suggests to them. They're having fun.

Contrary to what is portrayed in movies and literature, it is impossible to cause someone to do something that is against his morals or his principles while he is participating in hypnosis. If a suggestion were to be made that is contrary to any value that a person holds, the person would immediately revert to an alert state.

What many people may not know is that hypnosis is being used to benefit people in many medical, dental and therapeutic applications. Hypnosis is widely used to help people release fears, overcome the discomfort of the effects of chemotherapy, prepare for surgery, stop stuttering, end nail-biting and a host of other annoying habits. Hypnosis is so effective that it was recognised in 1957 by the

American Medical Association as a beneficial therapy for many physical and emotional needs. In the UK, the therapeutic benefits of hypnotherapy were acknowledged by the British Medical Association as early as 1892.

Hypnosis is a very natural state that most of us exist in during a large part of the day. When we become engrossed with our work and lose track of time or of what is going on around us, that is hypnosis. We are in a hypnotic state when we get caught up in daydreams or become so immersed in a movie or a television show that we emotionally react to what the actors are experiencing.

When you are in hypnosis during your labour, you'll be able to hear conversations and may, or may not, wish to join in. Though you will be totally relaxed, you will also be fully in control. To the person who is not familiar with self-hypnosis, you may even appear as though you've taken some kind of medication to put you into this profoundly relaxed state. During your birthing you will be aware of your uterine surges, but you will experience them comfortably, and with the knowledge that you are very much in charge. You'll be able to interrupt your relaxation whenever you wish and resume it whenever you wish.

As your labour moves nearer to birth, you will most likely choose to go even deeper within to your birthing body and your baby so that together you can work in harmony through birth. Though you will not be able to visually experience it, you will be able to physically know that your baby is very much a birth partner in this adventure. When you are tuned into your body, you will sense and know exactly what you and your baby are doing.

You'll become skilled in using your own natural abilities to bring your mind and body into perfect harmony. You will gain an understanding of the physiology of labour that goes beyond what is usually taught in other classes. You will learn special relaxation conditioning and labour techniques that will enable you to connect with and work with your body and your baby as you experience labour. The repetitive practise of these techniques will make it possible for you to instantly achieve this relaxation and maintain it for as long as you wish through labour.

The value of self-hypnosis comes from learning to reach that level of mind where suggestions that you give yourself effectively influence your physiological experience. Your HypnoBirthing practitioner will help you learn to reach this level, where you focus only on calm and comfort. You will see, hear and practise these techniques in class and will be given practise tapes or CDs that you will work with on a daily basis at home. Your birth companion will also be given scripts to use when you practise together two or three times a week.

There is no magic benefit that accrues from just coming to classes. You must be willing to apply the practise that is required to reach these levels of relaxation that will be there for you when you are in labour.

These skills will be applicable to many facets of your life, as well as for the birthing of your child. Many couples find that the months of preparation in relaxation benefit them in the way they deal with day-to-day situations and have a positive effect on how they interact with each other. A mum who was in one of my classes said, "I came to HypnoBirthing to learn how to have a baby, and I learned how to have a life". It's that powerful if you learn to utilise it.

Relaxation also has a calming effect upon the baby. "Mellow" is the word many parents use when describing their babies. We like to think they are "better natured".

Falling in Love with Your Baby

Leave it to a baby to turn your world upside down, take
your breath away and make you fall in love again. With his
toothless grin, your baby sets your heart on fire.

JAN BLAUSTONE, THE JOY OF PARENTHOOD

We know that calm, soothing thoughts and emotions have a bearing on the way in which you bring your baby into the world. Love
is one of the most important emotions in helping to build a positive
anticipation – the love that you as parents feel for each other and the
love that you actively share with the baby that you are carrying.

When is the best time for you to fall in love with your baby? If
you haven't already fallen madly in love with your baby and are not
playing and communicating with her on a daily basis, now is the
time. Getting acquainted with your baby is a very magical experience, and you don't have to wait until she is born to enjoy making
this connection.

Once your baby is born, you wouldn't think of going about
your daily routine without making time for frequent breaks that
are especially devoted to talking, playing and loving her. Babies
have a way of drawing that kind of attention from family members
and strangers alike. No one can resist their magnetic charm – so
compelling it can bring activities and conversation to a screeching
halt.

You can begin to connect socially and emotionally with your
unborn baby as soon as you know that you are pregnant. In addition
to making your pregnancy so much more enjoyable and exciting,
when you "tune in" to this little person who has become part of your
life, you lay the foundation for a relationship that can last for the

rest of your lives. Pre-birth parenting activities tell your baby that he is welcome and wanted.

The idea that both parents influence their pre-born baby is neither supposition nor superstition. The close bond that is built while the baby is still in the womb can be very real when it is time to connect with your baby during birthing.

Thanks to the relatively young study of foetology, advanced during the late seventies and early eighties by Dr. Thomas Verny in his book *The Secret Life of the Unborn Child*, we know that babies are cognizant during their time in the womb. In addition to developing physically, babies are developing mentally, emotionally and psychically. Parents should do all they can to be sure that the baby's emotional development, his sense of well-being and his esteem as a loved being are being fostered through caring and consistent pre-birth parenting.

The nine months that the baby spends in the womb are nine months of growth and development for parents as well. They learn the importance of evolving as a family, and mums learn the importance of planning and working, together with their babies, toward achieving the goal of a gentle birth for both baby and mother. Dr. David Chamberlain, author of *Babies Remember Birth*, later published as *The Mind of Your Newborn Baby*, spent many years investigating the effects of birth trauma upon a baby. He states that babies are active participants in birth, and they do remember their birth experience. The imprint of that experience is carried throughout their lives. All one has to do is gaze into the alert, knowing eyes of a newborn who has not been drugged during her journey into being, and it is immediately evident that there is a lot of thought going on. Without saying a word, the baby transmits a message: *I know.*

Antenatal and perinatal psychology is a branch of research that focuses on the effects of environment upon the baby as he is developing within the womb and during the birthing experience. Ongoing study is attempting to determine the degree to which a baby in the uterus is affected by the environment in which he is living and the manner in which his parents interact with him and each other.

While we know that everything the mother puts into her body crosses the placenta and affects the baby, this is also true of emotions. When we offer the pre-born baby love, play and music, we reinforce his positive feelings of security. On the negative side, it's been found that the pulse rate of the unborn baby rises abruptly when the baby is exposed to screaming, yelling, loud or disturbing noises and emotional upsets. Be aware of the kind of environment and experiences you are providing for your unborn baby.

It is so important that dads get involved in nurturing both mother and baby, and that mothers recognise the need for nurturing both dad and baby. Reciprocal nurturing of one parent for the other sends a strong message of security to their pre-born baby: This is a loving family.

As a result of Verny's studies, and those of his colleagues, it was found that babies in the womb react to stimuli outside of the uterus. Intentionally initiating certain kinds of interaction and love play can result in positive antenatal, perinatal and postnatal bonding.

Findings suggest that babies within the womb react to vibrations, stroking, tapping, rubbing, squeezing, conversation, voices, music, light, heat, cold, pressing to simulate the birth experience, teasing, loud noises, TV sounds and humour.

Babies who were exposed to soft music and singing during their time in the womb were calmer, happier and better adjusted to life outside of the womb. It is also believed that they are better sleepers. Babies love the sound of their parents' voices, especially when they are sung to. Some mothers report that while singing to their pre-born babies, the babies responded with a gentle moving action. Music has vibration that babies are sensitive to. If the vibration is gentle and calming, they have a feeling of well-being.

Dr. Michael Lazarev, a leading Russian paediatrician, noted that parents who interact with their unborn babies through music find a response from the baby. He emphasises the importance of helping the baby to become familiar with musical sounds, both before it is born and while it is an infant. Lazarev concluded that if you listen to your unborn baby, he will let you know what activities and sounds he prefers.

One Russian woman in the Lazarev study reported that when she was thirty-seven weeks pregnant, she attended a rock concert but had to leave because her baby was kicking in an agitated way so furiously that she felt she was going to be sick. Another mother reported that if she listened to Rachmaninoff and visualised swimming, the baby began to move in a soft, swirling manner. Another couple told of engaging in an argument. Their baby began to react in a way that let them know he wasn't comfortable with their tone. A woman who used to read fairy tales to her baby could sense by the kind of movement within the uterus that her baby was enjoying the stories.

In a study at the University of Salzburg, mothers who developed a real sense of being connected with their pre-born babies and who interacted with the babies in talk and play tended to view their bodies with an air of pride and fully accepted their increasing size as a natural part of the development of the baby. Fathers who were involved in bonding displayed the same kind of awe with respect to the shape of the mother's body and the development taking place inside. There was a respect for the life being carried in the womb. Overall, their pregnancies seemed to be easier, as were their birthings. They approached birthing with a relaxed confidence. Later, both parents seemed to adopt a softer, more balanced attitude toward caregiving. Parents displayed greater feelings of enjoyment, love and respect for each other and for the baby.

The benefits to babies were also profound. There were fewer premature births and fewer low-birthweight babies. Reports showed a noticeable increase in the socialisation of the babies who experienced pre-birth parenting. Overall health and weight gain were very positive. HypnoBirthing parents tell us that their young babies hardly cry and are exceptionally alert.

I believe that one of the most important advantages of pre-birth parenting to the baby is that when parents truly connect in attitude as a family prior to the birth of the baby, they accept the responsibility for planning and directing their births. They are as committed to ensuring the safety and comfort of the baby during its journey into the world as they are when their baby is part of their family outside the womb. I also believe that pre-birth parenting helps them become practised in accepting the responsibility of parenting later.

Chamberlain says that it is now widely known that babies actually develop their own physical exercise routine that is consistent throughout their life in the womb. Knowing that the baby is fully aware of its surroundings and the people who are his parents, it is only reasonable that the baby also thrives when there is interaction and socialisation with the people with whom he lives.

RECOMMENDATIONS FOR PRE-BIRTH PARENTING

- Learn the suggested relaxation techniques and practise them daily – baby needs peace, too. Since baby is aware, he is listening to the music and calming suggestions at the same time as his mum.
- Play with baby physically – sway, sway, sway; rub, rub, rub; pat, pat, pat; squeeze, squeeze, squeeze; press, press, press (all done gently).
- Use guided imagery and visualisation. (See the *Birth Companion's Reading* and *Rainbow Relaxation* in this book, as well as the Pre-Birth Parenting CD.)
- Carry on conversations with baby – say affirmations, read stories with animation and imitation of animal sounds, play children's tapes.
- While relaxing in the tub, massage your belly with lukewarm water and sing or talk to your baby.
- Play soothing music – sounds of ocean, birds, wind, soft piano, guitar, madrigals, flute, harp, nature sounds and animal sounds – so that baby develops a wider awareness of these things.
- Have family and friends greet and interact with baby.
- Put yourself in the baby's frame of reference – how wholesome are the surrounding noises, voices, attitudes, emotions, foods, temperatures, air, odours?

ANTENATAL BONDING EXERCISES

An important facet of the HypnoBirthing programme are the discussions and exercises for parents that help them to truly connect and fall in love with their pre-born baby. These activities help the parents develop a sensitivity to how the baby perceives his surroundings and often cause them to evaluate how their lifestyle, their emotional well-being, and their relationship with each other can impact the baby's emotional development and sense of feeling loved and secure.

The exercises on the HypnoBirthing Pre-Birth Parenting CD are valuable relaxation lessons and image-building tools for both parents. These activities help them develop a stronger sense of their own self-worth, as well as serve as meditations that will help them bond with their pre-born baby. The time spent with these guided images may prove to be among the most valuable gifts that you can give to yourself and your baby.

Another way to establish a connection with your baby and to explore his world is to take part in the following exercise. We call it "Be the Baby" because we ask you to imagine yourself in the role of the baby in the womb, experiencing what life is like for the baby.

As the practitioner leads you through this exercise, take advantage of the opportunity to think about how your unborn baby might respond to these questions, and how you can begin to actively do things that will enhance the baby's feeling of being loved and wanted.

BE THE BABY EXERCISE

What your baby perceives – what she accepts and embraces while in the uterus – becomes part of her essence and identity, and forms the creation of a conscious ego that accepts, caresses and acknowledges its own true self.

Imagine that you are the baby developing within your mother's womb, listening to conversations, experiencing your surroundings, absorbing emotions and moods of those around you. Reflect for a few minutes on how you feel as that child who will soon be born into your family.

- To what degree are your parents spending time in relaxation practise to help ensure a calm birth for you?
- How welcome do you feel? Do you already feel that you are part of the family?
- How loved do you feel? Do people talk to you with love each day?
- What kinds of messages are you receiving from things that are said about you?
- How do you feel about the way your parents interact with each other?
- What kind of pace do your parents keep? Do you feel sure there will be time purposely created for you as you're growing up?

- What kind of atmosphere will you come into? Peaceful? Loving? Caring? Happy?
- How confident are you that you will be raised with love and patience?
- How calm a world is being prepared for you?
- How kind and loving are the people you will be living with?
- Do you feel that your parents will do what is necessary to ensure your gentle entry into the world?
- Do your parents talk in gentle, loving ways?
- Is each motion that you make received with joy?
- What kinds of sounds/music/noises do you live with?
- Are you being provided with the best nourishing food to help you grow and develop in a strong, healthy way?
- How wholesome is the air that you are breathing? Will it foster good health for you?
- Is your environment and your body free of smoke, alcohol and drugs?
- How certain are you that you will be helped and guided toward becoming a loved and loving human being?
- What kind of assurance do you have that your parents will give you understanding as you learn to adjust to your strange, new world?
- Are you confident that you will learn by guidance, not punishment?

Reflecting on your responses to these questions, are there some changes that you feel you can make in your baby's environment? Are there some resolutions that you, as parents, need to think about and adopt?

We recommend these activities for creating lasting expressions of welcome for your baby:

- Write letters to the baby or keep a journal expressing your delight that he will soon be here. Save letters to present to the child later.
- Take pregnancy photographs of mother, as well as mother and dad together.
- Record messages to your baby on a tape or CD in addition to letters.

- Videotape your birthing, complete with a birthing-day message given to the baby during labour.
- Videotape siblings talking and listening to the baby or telling the baby a story.
- Involve siblings in decorating baby's room and take pictures.
- Start a scrapbook and include pictures that show how your body is changing as the baby develops, as well as special events like a visit from grandparents, trips to memorable places, a baby shower, a mother-baby luncheon, or a blessing way.

All natural birth has a purpose and a plan; who would think of tearing open the chrysalis as the butterfly is emerging? Who would break the shell to pull the chick out?

Selecting Your Caregivers and the Birthing Environment

Birth in a Sanctuary? Why not!

Imagine …
>   A place where everyone
>   Honours you and the work you will do in labour,
>   Speaks quietly and moves slowly and gently,
>   Respects your need to be spontaneous – to eat, drink make
>   sounds, move around, cry, shout, laugh,
>   Treats you and your baby as fully conscious and sensitive
>   beings.
>
>   Giving birth is as intimate as lovemaking
>   You will need privacy and support and tenderness
>   Labour is not a spectator sport
>   Your partner is not your "coach"
>   It's the journey of a lifetime for your baby and you
>   Don't settle for a typical birth
>   Find out more … home birth … birth centres
>   Safe alternatives to epidurals … Seek out a midwife
>   Arrange for a labour companion/doula to stay with you …
>   Protect your baby and empower yourself!

SUZANNE ARMS

SELECTING A CARE PROVIDER

Some of the decisions you both will make regarding your birthing may determine the birth memory that you and your baby will share forever.

In order to achieve the gentle birth that you are seeking, you will need to accept responsibility for choosing the right birthing environment – hospital birth, home birth, midwifery-led unit or birth centre.

Whether you are just beginning your pregnancy or are very near to the time when you will birth, your task right now is ensuring that the person or persons you invite, or have already invited, to be your birthing attendants share and support your view of birth, and that they will bring to your birthing the necessary understanding, care and patience to watch your birth unfold in a natural way. You can't leave it to chance, cross your fingers and hope that when your birthing time arrives, the caregiver who walks through the door of your birthing room will be on the same page of your Birth Preference Sheets as you are.

How do you go about choosing the right caregiver and the right environment? Think about other decisions you may have made in your life when choosing professionals and examine the strategies you took in making those final choices. If you were building a home, would you choose a building professional who has his own agenda – one who doesn't listen to you or consult with you about your feelings, opinions and ideas? Would you plan a holiday and not bother to learn anything about the hotel you will stay in? I'm sure the answer to all of these questions is an emphatic "No". And these are not possible life-changing decisions. Your baby's birth can be a life-changing event.

Preparing for your baby's birth is far more important than any other major decision you have ever made. You simply can't "settle". As one US HypnoBirther, Dr. Lome Campbell of New York, says, "Birth is the last frontier in woman's quest for freedom. A woman needs to be free to birth her babies as she chooses." You achieve that freedom only when you take responsibility for seeing that the people you surround yourself with are people who respect and support your dreams. You do have choices, and you need to identify them.

Begin your search with caregivers who are already on board with normal birthing. When you begin your education on care providers, don't limit it to well-intentioned friends who are passing on stories of their less-than-joyful birthings. You cannot risk taking their advice and hope that the interventionist caregiver whom they hired will be any less inclined to manage and control your labour with intervention and drugs.

Stringent educational requirements of health-care providers

assure you that most are equally qualified, but that doesn't mean that they all look upon birth in the same way. Just recently a doctor responded to the question, "Why did you choose obstetrics?" with the answer, "I've always been fascinated with surgery". Clearly, this doctor does not feel strongly that vaginal birth is natural and normal or even desirable. Her stated preference is for surgical birth. Her birth statistics would probably reflect her "fascination". This kind of information can and should be gleaned from your discussions during your interviews, not months later.

It is not uncommon for families to have no idea of where their caregiver stands on the management of labour until just before the baby is due to arrive or until the first suggestion of intervention is brought up. Whether you are just starting your search or if you are already familiar with your health-care provider, it is essential that you know what you can expect at the time of your birthing. These are subjects that need to be addressed.

As you talk with health-care providers, avoid sounding as though you are attempting to coerce or convert providers who don't look at birth in the same light as you. Your presence in their office is not to challenge a provider's views or to be confrontational. Be sure that your questions are framed in a polite and courteous way. The HypnoBirthing approach is not intended to do battle with the medical community or attempt to convert them. We do hope, of course, that once they have had the opportunity to see the calm of Hypno-Birthing, they will convert themselves.

One obstetrician became a convert to HypnoBirthing when many of her patients chose to birth their babies with our method. When it came time for her to birth her own first child, Dr. Patricia Calvo, a doctor in Fort Lauderdale, Florida, chose HypnoBirthing – a path that she never learned in medical school. Dr. Calvo believes that doctors should open themselves to gentle, relaxed methods, as long as they are safe. For her own birth, she said she had the best of both worlds.

Here are some helpful hints on finding the right health-care professional:

- Search until you find the provider who will honour your requests for no intrusive interventions to the same extent that he or she would accommodate couples who wish to utilize every bit of available technology and procedures.
- If you are already seeing a midwife or obstetrician, and you don't feel the degree of confidence that you think you should feel, speak up for yourself and your baby, and discuss your preferences early and often. If the discussion doesn't allay your doubts, be willing to seek the services of someone else who will give you that confidence.

One of the first things you should ask would be, "Are there midwives in the system I am currently using who are particularly open to natural birth?" You may want to spell out that what you mean by natural birth is birth without medication or intervention unless necessary. Some people now refer to natural birth as any birth that is not a surgical birth, regardless of the introduction of much intervention and medication. Many midwives are willing to cater to HypnoBirthing families and are happy to honour their wishes.

Dr. Wayne Goldner in Manchester, New Hampshire, was among the first obstetricians to witness a HypnoBirthing. Dr. Goldner has said, "I'll get up in the middle of the night, any day of the week, to attend this kind of birth." He and his associates do so on many occasions. They are patient and respectful of parents' wishes.

An obstetrician in Southern California, who took the HypnoBirthing Practitioner Certification workshop and embraces our philosophy of gentle birth, gives a silver spoon to every baby whose birth he attends. He believes that every baby should be born with a silver spoon in his mouth.

Also in Southern California, a doctor, who is a certified HypnoBirthing practitioner, encourages all her patients to use HypnoBirthing if they are able. Her practice is now so busy that she has to refer couples to another HypnoBirthing practitioner for their classes.

Another New Hampshire doctor often attends births sitting on the floor in front of a mother who chooses to birth on a birthing stool. He arranges for pillows to be put under the birthing stool so that the baby will be safe. He openly says that he doesn't do anything but watch. He attends births; he does not "deliver". He is a true example of one who lives by the root word for obstetrics – *obstare* – "to stand by".

His birth manner reminds me of the saying that likens a birth attendant to a lifeguard who is there to save a person from drowning, but who wouldn't think of rushing in to interfere with the person who is swimming perfectly well, lest in doing so he would interrupt the rhythm of the swimmer and perhaps cause him to panic and founder.

There are many similarly wonderful, gentle and caring birth attendants who love women, love babies and love birth. You should settle for nothing less.

Even in an ideal situation, you may need to keep reminding the caregiver that you are planning for a HypnoBirthing. Mention your birth preferences early and often, without being irksome. Health-care providers are busy people, who see many families. They sometimes need that gentle reminder.

If you've had a surgical birth previously and truly want to birth vaginally this time, seriously look into having a VBAC (vaginal birth after caesarean) and actively seek a doctor who will encourage you. The HypnoBirthing method is especially favorable to VBACs because the breathing techniques are gentle all through the opening phase, and you will not strain with forced pushing during the baby's descent – another plus for the VBAC mother.

Many providers who have never seen HypnoBirthing are more than happy to keep an open mind and support your wishes if they are presented to them in an inviting, rather than demanding, way. Many even enjoy being reminded why they chose to work in birthing before they got caught up in the "busy"ness of it all. They are there; you just need to find them.

YOUR OPTIONS – AND YOU DO HAVE CHOICES

There is no one system of care that covers the entire UK. Several systems are in place; but it is true to say that midwife-led care is the norm for most healthy, low-risk women in the National Health Service (NHS). Midwives are considered the guardians of normal birth and will do their utmost to see that normal birth is achieved. Their philosophy is sometimes shared with the general practitioner; but, for the most part, it is the midwife who is seen as the birthing expert.

The clientele of the midwife is mostly healthy women in a low-risk category. However, midwives are trained to detect possible abnormalities and make an appropriate referral to a doctor.

There are choices for midwifery services. When making your decision, look into your heart, consider your birthing wishes, and be sure that you feel comfortable with your choice. The following options are legitimate from both a safety and comfort perspective:

Community Midwives: Community midwives are organised into groups of six to eight midwives. Their services include antenatal appointments at clinics in the community, as well as home visits for anywhere from 10 to 29 days following the birth of the baby. Women working with community midwives may choose to give birth at home, and will have an opportunity, in most cases, to meet the group of midwives prior to their birthings.

A small percentage of women who choose to birth in the local hospital will be cared for by a team member, the others will be cared for by a staff midwife at the hospital.

The idea of team midwifery is popular with women preparing to give birth since they are able to get to know the person who will attend their birth and they are able to discuss their preferences beforehand. Midwives are guided by the women's choices for birthing and are equally comfortable giving support to a woman wishing a fully natural birth, as with a woman who feels that she may need some degree of medication.

Midwife-led Birth Centres: Another option in some areas is an NHS midwife-led birth centre. These units are made as homelike as possible. They have pools for labour and/or birthing and are staffed solely by midwives and health-care assistants or maternity-care assistants.

Independent Midwives: The concept of working with an independent midwife is also another option. Independent midwives are trained by the NHS and must practice by their standards. Most support natural birth and encourage the use of a birthing pool and homeopathy to enhance the experience.

You may hire an independent midwife by contacting the midwife and arranging a private agreement for her services. The agreement may be dependent upon whether all or only part of the care is to be covered by the midwife, and fees are charged accordingly. (For more information visit www.independentmidwives.org.uk.)

If your pregnancy is categorised as high risk, you will probably need to have a caregiver who attends births in the hospital. Midwives work in close conjunction with physicians in the event that a birthing does require a medical referral. Midwives usually are quite receptive to listening and supporting the wishes of birthing parents, but this, too, can differ with individuals.

My three recent trips to England to teach HypnoBirthing certification classes have allowed me to observe an entirely different approach to birth than what we experience in the United States. It is interesting to note the attitude toward midwifery and birthing in the United Kingdom and contrast it with ours in the United States. In the United Kingdom, midwives are the principal attendants at births and have a legal obligation to attend a birthing mother wherever she wishes to birth. In the early 1990s, the House of Commons in the UK officially mandated that the needs of birthing mothers be the central focus of maternal health-care providers and that maternity services be fashioned around them, not the other way around. Refreshing!

In the United Kingdom and other countries that operate under a National Health System (NHS), your birthing attendant could be one of any number of midwives. A midwife in the United Kingdom works with the NHS, serving women with normal pregnancies and labour.

In addition to doing all of the antenatal clinics and attending births, he/she will also cover the postnatal period up to twenty-eight days. While their clientele is mostly healthy women in a low-risk category, midwives are trained to detect possible abnormalities and make an appropriate referral to a doctor. Under this system, healthy women with healthy pregnancies can be attended by midwives, and most women never need to see a doctor. Almost three quarters of women birthing in the Netherlands are attended by midwives.

One of my mums had her first baby last Sunday at home. She completed the course with me only two weeks earlier. ... She went into labour spontaneously and called the homebirth midwife to come and check her because she was "getting some strange sensations"! The midwife stayed for an hour and concluded that there was no way the mum was in active labour. The midwife could not tell when the mum was having surges and had to ask her to indicate them by squeezing her husband's hand so that the baby could be monitored.

Baby and mother were so calm that the midwife said that she would leave them for a few hours and to call if things progressed. The mum then said, "Before you go, can you just tell me – is it normal to want to push at this stage?" The midwife was compelled to do an examination and found that the mum was fully open and the head was visible!! A beautiful baby boy was breathed into the world twenty minutes later.

Later, as the midwife was leaving, she said to a very ecstatic, proud and alert mum, "Well, I have never seen anything like that before. You are obviously made to have babies." To which the mum replied: "Yes, I'm a woman!"

VANESSA, WALES, U.K.

In some areas, you may have the option of a midwifery system called the Domino scheme, whereby community midwives are attached to a hospital. The Domino scheme provides the same continuity of care as for a home birth, but provides the opportunity for a woman to give birth in hospital, if she feels that is where she will be most comfortable. This option can mean that all antenatal services will be conducted by midwives, with the possibility of seeing a different midwife at each visit. If your labour is prolonged or spills from one shift to another, you could have more than one midwife attend your birthing.

I was in my fortieth week of pregnancy and had looked forward to a planned homebirth, but a late test result indicated that it couldn't be. I needed to change plans fast for birthing with a midwife and seek a physician. I felt this would not be an easy task at this late date.

I called my family physician, Dr. Barrett, and made an appointment to see him on Friday morning. The man earned high honours in my book for being willing to take me on as a patient at exactly forty weeks. I knew him to be a wonderful doctor and a very compassionate man.

Friday afternoon, I began to have surges. This was nothing new to me, as I had had surges off and on for many weeks, but these were two to three minutes apart and felt different. We got packed, got into the car and headed for the hospital.

We arrived a little after 3:30 and were admitted. Much to my delight, the surges continued to get longer and stronger. Our doula, Missy, showed up soon after. Our nurse was puzzled that I could walk, talk and smile through surges, and seemed flustered to think that I was going to birth without an epidural. She said that unless the cervix is changing, it isn't real labour. I'm sure that she didn't believe that I was in true labour – too quiet and too relaxed. She called Dr. Barrett when I declined to answer the questions on the pain scale and told him that I had a very bossy doula who was telling me that I could refuse things. He supported my position.

When my membranes released at 6:40, I began to feel pressure. Missy recognised the signs and felt that this was going to be a really short labour. Reluctantly the nurse called Dr. Barrett. As soon as he came into the room, I released and began to nudge the baby down. Two surges later, our baby was born. I held him in my arms and cried with happiness for love of him and relief that he was here, alive and healthy.

Dr. Barrett spent the next two hours with us, as did Missy. He personally secured warm blankets for me, made sure I had food, gave me his pager number and did all the sweet things you would expect from a good friend. He was supportive of all the things I wanted. I gave birth without an IV or medication, ate throughout labour and had no anaesthesia.

This birth was different from what I had envisioned and hoped for a few weeks earlier, but it was the birth that our baby needed, and a beautiful birth at that.

MELANIE, SALT LAKE CITY

Obstetrician: Obstetricians are medical doctors who have graduated from an accredited school of medicine and have completed two to three years of advanced study in the field of gynaecology and obstetrics. They are highly trained surgeons and are proficient at detecting, diagnosing and treating gynaecological and obstetrical problems that require specialised procedures. They are skilled specialists who are called upon when special circumstances arise in birthing that require specific medical or surgical procedures. Because they are prepared and trained for surgical births, they would be most likely to see a large number of mothers who are in the category of high risk.

Obstetricians see pregnant women for examinations, testing and other antenatal care, as well as postnatal checkups. If a surgical birth is deemed necessary, an obstetrician will perform the caesarean section. Obstetricians do not need backup from another surgeon, except in rare or unusual circumstances.

I was concerned that I might not find a doctor who would understand our wanting to birth naturally, but Dr. Adams was wonderful. He had never heard of HypnoBirthing, but asked if he could take our book home with him to share with his wife who is preparing to become a doula. He was very accepting of our birth preferences.

My "Guess Date" was May 6, and on May 11, with my blood pressure rising, our doctor suggested induction. I was already at 4 centimetres open, and he knew that labour was near.

We arrived at the hospital at 7:00 the following morning. Dr. Adams said that he would rupture the membranes rather than give me something stronger.

We spent the day walking when I wasn't being monitored. My husband said that I looked like I was drugged because I was so relaxed. When a surge came, I simply stopped walking and talking and closed my eyes. I visualised waves rolling in and out on a beach.

I was 6 centimetres opened at 6:00 P.M., but I wasn't told what stage I was in. I didn't want to know.

At 7:00 P.M., I felt I needed to be checked. I asked the nurse not to tell me how open I was because I didn't want to be disappointed or to ruin my frame of mind. She checked and said, "Well, I'll say this. I need to call the doctor and tell him to come quickly." Our baby was on his way down. When I crowned, I pushed two or three times, and my baby was born. I had an eight-pound baby boy at 8:36 P.M.

Throughout the whole birthing, I felt about one second of pain. I was scared by the sensation of tearing. I had two tiny tears that healed in a couple of days.

I did not need to practise time distortion because the whole day was a blur. I couldn't believe that twelve hours had passed. Our doctor and the nurses were truly amazed.

Our baby is easygoing, a good sleeper and nurses well, which I attribute to his calm, drug-free birth.

Thanks to a supportive doctor and to our HypnoBirthing practitioner for a miracle to be treasured always.

TERESA, VERMONT

Here are a few questions you might ask the person(s) you are considering selecting to get a feel for their openness to normal birthing:

- We are planning to do HypnoBirthing – a natural birth; will you support us in that?
- How often do you perform caesarean births? What is the most common reason?
- Considering ten of your patients, how many do you feel will need to be induced? Need augmentation? Have a caesarean section?
- If our baby is strong, and I am fine, will you postpone discussion of induction until forty-two weeks?
- If release of membranes is the first sign of labour, how long are you willing to wait for spontaneous onset of labour? Why do you choose that number?
- During the birthing phase, I will be breathing the baby down to birth rather than forcefully pushing. Are you comfortable with that?
- I would like to eat light snacks for energy while in labour. What is your feeling about that?

Professional Labour Companion/Doula: A professional labour companion (PLC) is a person who knows birthing and, from behind the scenes, helps parents achieve the uninterrupted birth they are seeking. A PLC frees the birth companion to focus his or her attention upon the mum, while the PLC tends to details of seeing that the mum has a cool facecloth that is refreshed regularly and reminds her to change positions or to empty her bladder. One of the most important roles that a labour companion plays is that of liaison with hospital staff when parents have a request or need help interpreting the situation. Just the presence of a labour companion helps to avoid the suggestion of intervention and allows parents to relax in the confidence that they are in good hands. (For more information on hiring a doula, visit www.doula.org.uk.)

CHOOSING YOUR BIRTHING ENVIRONMENT

In-Hospital Birth Centres: Some hospitals have an entire unit devoted to birthing and the care of newborn babies – these are midwifery-led units. They have discarded the old "Labour and Delivery" signs and replaced them with names that indicate a softer, less medicalised atmosphere. A great deal of money and effort have been put into making these units appear attractive, comfortable and homelike. This is very appealing, but you must evaluate more than the decor. Matching draperies and spreads give an air of charm and a homelike appearance, but unless the people who come into this setting to attend the birthing families have a matching attitude of kindness, are family-oriented and view birth as normal, the decor becomes only window dressing, disguising the equipment, instruments and machinery that may be in full force during your birthing.

Supporting the belief that healthy women with healthy babies can safely birth outside the "geared-for-emergency" protocol, there are hospitals that are truly committed to natural birthing and family-friendly care and attention. Some of them have even allocated a sizeable segment of the birthing unit, and in some cases an entire floor, to families who want to birth naturally. These rooms are free of monitors and other medical equipment and apparatus. Mums are not immediately stripped of their clothing, put to bed, strapped to a machine and outfitted with an IV. Staff members are carefully selected to support the families who choose to birth there.

A hospital in Rochester, New Hampshire, is so committed to gentle birth that nearly half of all of their births are HypnoBirthings. Thanks to the efforts of caring nurses and administrators, as well as the goodwill of a few HypnoBirthing practitioners, a hospital in San Diego, California, has an entire floor devoted to families who want to birth in an atmosphere that is as close to normal as possible. A large hospital in Chicago has an ABC unit (Alternative Birth Centre), as do many others across the country. The trend is growing. You will want to be sure that the hospital you select is truly HypnoBirthing-friendly, lending an atmosphere that says birth is normal and not an emergency waiting to happen.

William and Martha Sears, authors of *The Birth Book*, suggest that "parent power" is the answer to making care providers and hospital administrators more sensitive to this need. When millions of expectant families call the hospital of their choice and ask for such accommodations, including a staff that supports normal birth, it will happen. Parents need to be aware, however, that, on occasion, the same hospital that teaches gentle birthing in their childbirth classes may meet the couple with "routine" procedures when they arrive at the hospital to birth their baby. Parents need to address this inconsistency, and it is a good idea to set the stage early. Ask the caregivers and the hospital staff, as well as parents who have birthed in that facility, if the facility is family-friendly and endorses the belief of normal birth.

If possible, tour more than one birthing facility and talk with the staff, just as you did when you selected your medical care provider. The answers to these questions will tell you about the hospital's philosophy. It's a good idea to do this early: You may want to change your plans based on your findings. Don't wait until just before your birthing time to inquire about these things.

Here are some questions for you to consider:

- Is there flexibility in policies and willingness to accommodate HypnoBirthing preferences in the absence of special circumstances?
- Are there midwives on staff who are partial to natural birth?
- Do they have a pool?
- Do they have birthing balls or can you bring one?
- Will you be fed if your labour lingers? Are snacks available?
- Are you free to walk outside or within the hospital?
- May you remain in your own clothes during labour?
- Is immediate, skin-to-skin bonding time allowed with the baby?
- Are labour companions/doulas welcome?
- Is there a provision for the partner and baby to stay in the same room as the mum?
- Are statistics on inductions, augmentations, epidurals and caesarean births available?

Free-standing Birth Centres: The birth centre is more likely to afford you the opportunity to birth without intervention. You will want to ask the same questions of a birth centre staff member as you do of hospital staff. Because the birth centre focus is on healthy

women with healthy pregnancies, they don't have to be equipped
with all of the high-tech apparatus that is needed for women with
pregnancy complications. Birthing in a birth centre, however, is as
safe as hospital birthing.

Homebirth: There is much misunderstanding and misinformation
about homebirths. Among them are the myths that homebirthing is
dangerous while hospital births are safe.

A study done by Dr. Lewis Mehl-Madronna in 1976, in conjunction with researchers at Stanford University, compared the
safety of homebirth with hospital births. The results showed that
morbidity outcomes of the 2,092 births studied were identical. The
study also showed that only 5 per cent of the mothers birthing at
home received medication, whereas 75 per cent of the in-hospital
births received medication. Even more revealing, three times as
many caesarean sections were performed on the mother in hospital
births as there were in the planned homebirths that required transfer to a hospital. Babies born in hospitals suffered more foetal
distress, newborn infection and birth injuries than did those born in
homes. Interestingly, 66 per cent of the homebirths were attended
by doctors, which would suggest that when women are relaxed in
the comfort of their own homes and are allowed to birth normally,
what is looked upon as a medical incident can evolve into something quite natural and safe.

Also, not commonly known is that the community midwife who
attends homebirths is required to carry the same equipment and
drugs that are used to meet the most common special circumstances
that occur in hospitals, although their need for it is very rare.

Baby's Choice: Occasionally, while their parents have plans that are
quite different, HypnoBirthing babies may decide that it is all right
to be born en route to the hospital or even in the comfort of their
own homes.

It is important to know that there is nothing about this situation
that creates an emergency or that is necessarily cause for panic. As
many taxi drivers and policemen will attest, babies can be born
safely wherever they choose. Should your baby decide that your
bedroom or the backseat of your car, away from the hustle and
bustle of other people, is perfectly fine with him, you can remain

calm and offer the same gentle birth you had planned earlier.

We suggest that when you set out for the hospital, drape the backseat of your car with plastic bags underneath a sheet, and be sure to bring pillows. It is better to pull over to the side of the road than to risk rushing through traffic. If you are at home, it is better to just get off your feet with something underneath you and relax where you are in your home than to risk having the baby emerge while you're running to get to the car. Baby will be much happier, and you will be better able to maintain the calm and joy of his birthing.

Since much of the apprehension over an unplanned out-of-hospital birth lies in questions about how to handle the umbilical cord, it is important for you to know that leaving the cord attached, even for hours, as is done in some cultures, is safe and quite beneficial to the baby. Your practitioner can offer more details.

Preparing Your Mind and Body for Success

> Muscles send messages to each other. Clenched fists, a tight
> mouth, a furrowed brow, all send signals to the birth-passage
> muscles, the very ones that need to be loosened. Opening
> up to relax these upper-body parts relaxes the lower ones.
>
> WILLIAM SEARS AND MARTHA SEARS

Most athletes will readily advise that relaxation and visualisation are crucial to successful performance. Golfers quickly learn not to "press", but to release and let go. It is not uncommon to see Olympic athletes standing off to the side running visualisations of their perfect performance through their minds. Sports greats know that stress and tension in the mind equate to stress and tension in the body; the two cannot be separated. Conquering stress and fear is what allows sports figures to appear to perform so effortlessly. It's impressive.

Also awe-inspiring is the serene look on the face of the HypnoBirthing mum as she experiences uterine surges. Equally impressive is the smile that creeps onto her face as she alerts herself following each surge. That smile has become a hallmark. There is no trace of exhaustion or dread as her gaze meets that of her birthing companion. The Sleep Breathing and Slow Breathing techniques learned in HypnoBirthing classes are the centrepiece of the HypnoBirthing programme. They help the birthing mother to be in touch with her own natural instincts – to let her body and her baby take over, while she experiences this wonderful event on a deeper level. Now is the time to train your mind and your body to naturally and instinctively do exactly what they need to do.

There are four basic techniques that we will cover in this section:

breathing, relaxation, visualisation and deepening. Each technique has several alternatives from which you can choose the one (or more) that you find most effective for you and that you like best. Learning to use all four techniques so that they become second nature to you will prepare your body and mind for the birth process.

THE FOUR BASIC HYPNOBIRTHING TECHNIQUES

Breathing	Visualization
Relaxation	Deepening

Taking the time to practise these techniques should be an essential part of your daily routine. There is absolutely no substitute for the work of this course in conditioning your mind and body in preparation for birth. You cannot simply attend classes and hope that the conditioning will occur without your dedication to making it happen. Conditioning involves your mind *and* your body. A skier would never attempt to compete in a tournament unless his body was conditioned. A runner would never attempt to enter a marathon unless his body was conditioned.

While birthing should not be the exhausting, pushing-your-body-to-the-edge feat that athletes face, it nevertheless requires the same kind of discipline so that when the time comes, you are ready. Since you are conditioning your mind for ultimate relaxation, it is important that you form a pattern that your mind can automatically respond to when it comes time for your birthing. It is time well spent, and it can cut the time and the effort you will spend in your labour. As one who has been there, I can emphatically say that conditioning is a *must*. You can't slough it off and hope that you'll get lucky.

YOUR RELAXATION PROGRAMME

One of the most effective tools for dealing with tension, stress and discomfort without drugs is your own conditioned ability to slip into relaxation and visualisation quickly and at any given moment. In HypnoBirthing you will learn relaxation techniques and visualisations that will see you through your labour and quickly bring about a renewed state of energy following your birthing. It is important that you rehearse these techniques so that you can call them up readily when they are needed.

ESTABLISHING YOUR ROUTINE

- Select a time to relax when you won't be disturbed. Take the receiver off the phone or turn off the ringer and answering machine.
- Set aside the same time each day and dedicate yourself to that time.
- Choose a comfortable practise spot that has soft, dim light and make that the place you will use daily.
- Be sure that your bladder is empty.
- Wear clothes that are not binding and use a soft throw over your body to ensure that you are comfortably warm.
- Use HypnoBirthing tapes or CDs. The background music tape consists of tones and rhythms that the body responds to best.

POSITIONS FOR RELAXATION

Your body is the best source of information on the position you will assume when doing relaxation with your tapes. The general rule is to use the position in which you feel most comfortable. The two recommended positions are:

BACK POSITION

Early in your pregnancy, you will no doubt be comfortable on your back while you practise relaxation. Later in your pregnancy, you will want to elevate your upper body to accommodate the extra weight of the baby. Once you gain more weight, you may choose to use a different position. If you are lying flat, the pressure of the weight of your baby can block the main blood vessel in your back, the inferior vena cava, and shut off the supply of blood and oxygen to the lower part of your body and your baby.

- If you choose to lie on your back, place pillows under your head and shoulders or use a large rolled towel or a pillow under your right side.

- Let your arms rest at your sides; bend elbows slightly and turn your shoulders down and outward, as though they were sinking into the cushion or pillow beneath you.
- Hands should be gently and softly cupped, palms downward and fingers resting in a rounded position on a flat surface at your side.
- Feet should be about six inches apart, turned outward, relaxed.

LATERAL POSITION

The lateral position is chosen most often by birthing mothers during late labour and frequently for birthing their babies. It is also a position that is usually assumed for sleeping during pregnancy.

- Lie on your left side with the left shoulder, neck and left side of the head resting on a pillow. The left arm should be placed loosely by your left side.
- With the elbow bent, rest the right arm to the side of the pillow.
- The left leg should be straight down, with the knee slightly bent.
- Bend the right leg up, placing the knee even with your hip with one or two pillows under the knee for support.

As you continue to work with the exercises for relaxation, you'll find that each one gives you an explanation of the benefits of the exercise

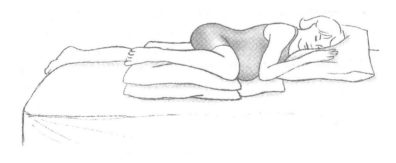

Lateral Position

and a brief script that you can use in practise with your birth companion. As you practise these recommended exercises, you will naturally find the one or ones that feel most comfortable for you. It is not necessary that you work with all of them. It is more important that you work with the technique that works best for you.

FACIAL RELAXATION

Achieving deep facial relaxation is most important as it will set the tone for the rest of your body. The lower jaw area directly affects the vaginal opening. When your lower jaw is relaxed, the vaginal area will also be relaxed. When you have mastered the art of facial relaxation, your jaws will be totally relaxed, with the-lower jaw slightly receded. You will be able to bring yourself into a natural state of relaxation instantly.

Technique

Let your eyelids slowly close. Don't try to force them shut. Just let them gently meet. Place your awareness on the muscles in and around your eyes. As you feel a natural drooping of the eye muscles, sense relaxation spreading from your forehead, down across your eyelids, over your cheekbones and around your jaws. Let your lower jaw recede as your teeth part. Your eyelids will feel heavier as your cheeks and your jaw go limp. Bring the relaxation within your eyes to a level where it seems as though your eyelids just refuse to work. Place the tip of your tongue at your palate where your upper teeth and palate meet, bringing about a sense of peace and well-being as you connect with an energy orbit in your body. Feel your head making a dent into your pillow. As you practise this technique, you will feel your neck, shoulders and elbows droop. Picture your shoulders opening outward and sinking down into the frame of your body as you go deeply into relaxation.

Breathing Techniques

There are only three gentle breathing techniques used in Hypno-Birthing. The first, Sleep Breathing, is simply a relaxation technique designed to help you enter a relaxed state so that you can continue with imagery and visualisation practise.

The second breathing technique is called Slow Breathing. This breathing style is most important as it is the breathing that you will use throughout the thinning and opening phase of your birthing when you experience a uterine surge.

The third style of breathing is called Birth Breathing. It's the technique that you will use during birthing when you are breathing your baby down through the birth path to emergence during the birthing phase. Unlike the other breathing styles, you will not actively practise Birth Breathing until the time you are almost ready to birth your baby, but it will be reviewed in detail when we handle the information on birthing.

SLEEP BREATHING

Oxygen is the most important fuel for the working muscles in the uterus. Your baby also needs to have a sufficient, continual supply of oxygen. That is why proper breathing is so important to your relaxation. The Sleep Breathing technique is used at the beginning of each relaxation practise to help your body gradually slip into a comfortable state of relaxation. You will want to focus your awareness on this technique early in your programme.

Sleep Breathing will help you to achieve relaxation when you are practising alone or with your birth companion. It is also one of the methods you will use to resume relaxation between uterine surges during birthing. This technique will help you to conserve energy during the thinning and opening phase of labour. For deep comfort, and to keep your body loose and limp, roll or fold a pillow under your knees so hips, joints and knees will be slightly bent. Allow your shoulders to open outward and sink into the frame of your relaxing body.

To establish a proper breathing technique for Sleep Breathing, practise the following exercise.

TECHNIQUE

Just relax and settle into the comfort of the chair or sofa beneath you and let the pillows behind you support your head and neck. Now allow your head to gently lean forward toward your chest or let it rest back onto the pillows behind you.

Let your eyelids gently meet without forcing them shut. Your mouth should be softly closed with your lips touching lightly. Place the tip of your tongue at your palate where your teeth and your palate meet and feel the wonderful sense of relaxation drifting throughout your body.

Draw in a breath from your stomach. To a count of four, mentally recite "In–2–3–4" on the intake. Feel your stomach rise as you draw the breath up and into the back of your throat.

As you exhale, mentally recite "Out–2–3–4–5–6–7–8". Do not exhale through your mouth. As you breathe out very slowly through your nose, direct the energy of the breath down and inward toward the back of your throat, allowing your shoulders to droop into the frame of your body. Breathe your body down into relaxation. Release all tension and let go.

To determine if you are doing this exercise correctly, place your left hand on your stomach and your right hand on the lower part of your chest. As you inhale, you should feel your left hand rising as though your stomach were inflating like a balloon. As you exhale, you will feel your hands fold into each other, as your chest and stomach create a crevice.

Sleep Breathing is easy to master. You will use it regularly in your classes and in your home practise. You'll feel relaxation coming more easily and rapidly each time you do it. When you have mastered the concept, it will not be necessary for you to recite numbers or test with your hands to guide yourself into this state. After only a few times, you will be able to bring your body into a deep state of relaxation in preparation for further deepening work.

SLOW BREATHING

Slow Breathing involves a long, quiet, slow intake of breath from your abdomen that redirects your focus to what is happening around your baby and helps you work with each surge. It takes practise and MUST be worked on daily. A few minutes when you awaken in the morning and before you fall asleep at night should provide you ample practise.

The goal of Slow Breathing is to make your breath, both in and out, as long as possible. You will use this technique through labour to coincide with each surge.

As indicated in the illustration below, when your uterus surges, it rises. Slow Breathing helps you to work in concert with that upward movement of the uterus as you breathe your abdomen up to the highest possible height – like filling an inner balloon. This maximises the wave of the vertical muscles, causing them to work more efficiently in drawing up the lower circular muscles, and thinning and opening the cervix. The assist that this gives to both sets of muscles shortens the length of the surge, as well as the length of labour.

When you first practise this breathing pattern, you will learn that its name indicates the manner of intake – long, *slow* breaths.

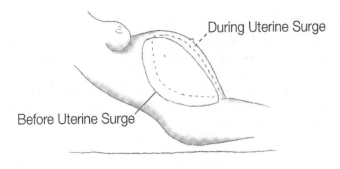

During Uterine Surge

Before Uterine Surge

The Uterus During Surge

The Uterus During Surge

TECHNIQUE

While resting your back against pillows or lying in a lateral position, place your hands across the top of your abdomen so that your fingers barely meet. Exhale briefly to clear your lungs and nasal passages. *Slowly* and gradually draw in your breath to a *rapid* count from 1 to 20+, as though you were inflating your belly. **Avoid using short intakes of breath;** it can tire you and requires that you take several breaths in order to get through the surge. The slow intake to a rapid count up to 20+ and the equally slow exhalation will allow you sufficient time to work with each surge. If it is necessary for you to take a second breath during a surge, do so in the very same manner. Do not hold your breath – ever.

Keep your body still and limp – NOT STIFF – and visualise your abdomen as being similar to a crater or a bowl in which your baby is resting. The rest of your body beneath the crater is totally relaxed and still while you breathe up each surge.

While breathing in, focus your attention on your rising abdomen and bring the surge up as much as you can; visualise filling a balloon inside your abdomen as you draw in. *Slowly* exhale to the same count, breathing downward and outward. Visualise the balloon slowly drifting off into space. Give your breath to your baby, gently and slowly exhaling down into your vagina.

You may find at first that you will reach an intake count of only 13 to 15. This is not unusual. You'll stretch the count more each time you do this exercise, and your count will rapidly increase to the long, slow intake. Regardless of how high a count you achieve, the technique of fully expanding the abdomen will be with you when you need it for labour. As each surge occurs, you will feel the results of your practise, taking in appropriately long, drawn-out breaths and equally long exhalations.

As with Sleep Breathing, once you have mastered the concept and the technique, you will not need to use numbers unless you prefer to keep pacing yourself to increase the count.

BIRTH BREATHING

Birth Breathing is used when you are breathing your baby down during the birthing phase of labour. It is intended to assist the Natural Expulsive Reflex (NER) of your body to move your baby gently down to crowning and birth.

Birth Breathing is NOT pushing. Pushing can be counterproductive and actually slow down the birthing process. The concept of forced breathing is totally invalid today. It stems from an earlier time when women were generally anaesthetised and unable to birth their babies. Forceps were employed to extract the baby from the vagina. When natural childbirth became popular in the late 1960s and early '70s, women for the first time in many generations were awake, and the use of forceps dwindled. It was then thought, however, that since there was no means of extracting the baby with instruments, the baby would have to be "pushed" down through the birth path and out past the vaginal outlet. Counted breaths of 1 and 2 and 3, all the way up to 10 – called "purple pushing" because the blood vessels in the mother's face and eyes become purple from the violent pushing – became the rule of the day.

Forced pushing creates stress for the birthing mother, which is self-defeating in that it closes the sphincters of the vagina ahead of the descending baby. Any woman who attempts to simulate forced pushing will immediately verify that there is a tensing of the muscles in the lower birth path, not a release.

There has been much written about the inefficiency of forced pushing and the possible damaging effect it has on the muscles of the birthing woman's pelvic floor, but it remains a necessary part of emergence in the minds of many caregivers and women themselves. While women who find themselves unable to push because of having had epidurals are allowed to "labour down" by letting their bodies naturally expel their babies, the woman in the next room who is birthing naturally is expected to forcefully "push her baby out". It is an unnecessary carryover when we consider that women in comas have given birth undetected.

With Birth Breathing, there is no need for a lengthy period of hard, violent pushing during descent. Your baby's descent will be gradual, but it will not necessarily take longer. The natural pulsations of your body will move your baby down the birth path efficiently and gently. Many mums report using only two or three Birth Breaths to bring their babies to full emergence. That's because the sphincters at the outlet are not tense and closed. The relaxed body will naturally open for you. Birth Breathing also gives your baby the advantage of a kinder and safer birth.

Forced pushing can exhaust you and press your baby against a resistant passage that is not yet receptive to his journey. Stories of exhaustive pushing that extends over hours bear out the fact that the baby will descend when he and the birth path are ready. There is no need to rush. Would we pull a butterfly from its chrysalis? The natural birthing process has a purpose that must be respected and trusted.

Often women themselves will speak of an overwhelming urge to push taking over. If this is felt, it is also because of conditioning that stems from a deeply embedded notion that babies cannot descend on their own. We seem to be the only mammals who turn our birthings into what appears to be a gymnastic event, complete with "squat bars" and knotted ropes on which mothers can suspend themselves. This scene hardly holds a mirror up to nature. Our animal sisters elect to gently expel their babies.

A calm, gentle nudging breath can be recaptured by slowly establishing the same kind of relaxation that you used for your Sleep Breathing practise. Even if you initially feel the conditioned "urge to push", surrendering to this impulse can totally turn your birthing around as it limits the amount of oxygen going to your baby. This can cause concern on the part of caregivers, as your baby's heart rate can decelerate. It may lead to the very special circumstance that you've worked so hard to avoid. Let your baby and your body determine the pace. Breathe down into your body to relax the vaginal outlet and follow whatever lead your baby takes.

Because Birth Breathing is not one of the techniques that you will practise routinely to prepare your body for birth, we will defer the directions for this breathing technique until later in the course when we go more thoroughly into the birthing process. It is helpful, though, to consider here the rationale for Birth Breathing and contrast it with strained and forced staff-directed breathing.

Let's consider the effect of each of the birthing styles:

Mother-Directed Birth Breathing	Staff-Directed Forced Pushing
Allows parents to maintain control over their birthing	Tires mother and reduces her effectiveness and participation in birthing experience
Conserves mother's energy	Closes and constricts vaginal passage ahead of baby
Provides continual supply of oxygen to the baby	Emergency intervention can result. Mother becomes exhausted; baby is distressed
Gently opens the birth path for smooth descent	Ruptures eye and facial blood vessels
Increases prospect of birthing over an intact perineum	Limits flow of oxygen to baby, often causing heart-rate deceleration
Perineal tissues unfold naturally for the gentle emergence of baby	Surrenders control of birthing to others
Baby maintains healthy heart-rate during descent	Contributes to tearing or the need for episiotomy

A pregnant woman is like a beautiful flowering tree, but take care when it comes time for the harvest that you do not shake or bruise the tree, for in doing so, you may harm both the tree and its fruit.

PETER JACKSON, R.N.

Relaxation Techniques

Once you have learned to bring your breathing into a smooth, rhythmic pace and you can ease yourself into relaxation effortlessly, you can then learn to bring your relaxation on instantly by using one of the methods included here. You do not need to master all of these techniques. You will naturally turn to the ones that are most effective for you and that you like best.

PROGRESSIVE RELAXATION

Sitting in a comfortable chair or sofa, associate each of the designated parts of your body from the top of your head to your toes with the number that corresponds to it on the illustration that follows. Take a deep breath, then as you exhale let it all instantly flow down through your body, causing your muscles to go totally limp. We refer to this state as "Lucy Limp" (Loosey Limp), the name of a soft doll that is like a Beanie Baby.

Eventually, you will be able to take one deep breath and rapidly count off the numbers as you exhale, bringing those parts of your body immediately into a limp state. The more rapidly you think the numbers, the more rapidly you will feel the effects. In using this practice, you should let your body go absolutely limp from the top to your toes. Let your head hang loose and forward, and let your arms and hands fall limp down by your side.

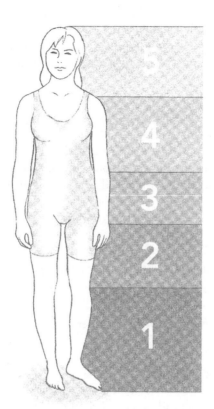

DISAPPEARING LETTERS

A similar technique for bringing yourself into a deep level of relaxation is to use the Disappearing Letters exercise. It is perhaps the easiest of all the instant relaxation techniques that you will use. It is especially helpful if you feel stressed during the day at work or home or if you need some help falling asleep. When using this technique as an aid to falling asleep, you will actually feel your head creating a deeper indentation into your pillow as your neck muscles thoroughly relax.

   With practise, you will find that by the time you reach the first or second "C", the rest of the letters of the alphabet will be erased from your mind. It will be too much effort to say or think the letters, and your body will be limp, as described earlier. This exercise is one of the fastest ways to bring yourself into a wonderful, comfortable state at any time. I recommend it especially to maintain a feeling of calm during that period of adjustment after your baby is born.

TECHNIQUE

- Close your eyes.
- Take in a quick, deep breath – pause.
- Quickly visualise the letters rolling by or coming forward and mentally say to yourself quickly while you exhale:

AAA–BBB–CCC–D ... etc.

- Allow your head, neck, shoulders and upper torso to instantly sink into the frame of your body. Give yourself permission to let your arms, hands and legs hang loosely. This can be accomplished in seconds and will be very useful for you when you are birthing, as well as at other times.

LIGHT TOUCH MASSAGE

Birth companions are taught the art of applying Light Touch Massage, a technique developed by Constance Palinsky of Michigan, after much research into pain management and the release of endorphins.

The theory of Light Touch is that the smooth muscle just below the surface of the skin, called *erector pili*, reacts by contracting when stimulated. When this occurs, the muscle pulls up the surface hair, which becomes erect and causes goose bumps. The goose bumps, in turn, help to create endorphins, those feel-good hormones that promote relaxation.

We use Light Touch Massage in birthing because when endorphins are secreted, catecholamine is not. The technique is very simple, yet effective. It is a wonderful comfort measure that the birthing companion brings to the labour room and as a means of nurturing during pregnancy. It is a great way for couples to feel physically closer to each other in the later stages of pregnancy.

The creation of endorphins resulting from practising Light Touch

Massage helps to keep our mums calm and comfortable, both prior to birthing and while in labour.

If, while the birth companion is applying Light Touch, he extends his hands out and around the sides of the breasts and nipples to apply light nipple stimulation, not only are endorphins produced, but also the hormone oxytocin, which naturally enhances uterine surges. For that reason, until you are approaching the very end of your term, the birth companion should *not* massage the nipples when practising this technique.

Light Touch Massage can be applied while the mum is sitting on a birth ball leaning on pillows at the side of a bed. If the couple is in a hospital, they can request that the foot of the bed be adjusted to create a kneeler. If birthing is taking place at home or in a birthing centre, the same effect can be achieved by kneeling on a pillow in front of a chair, a sofa or at the side of a bed with pillows stacked upright for you to rest your arms and head on. Your birthing companion can kneel behind you while administering Light Touch Massage as illustrated or can also use a chair.

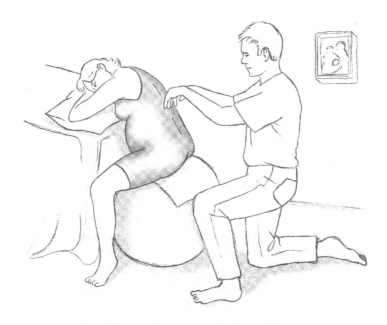

Birth Companion Applies Light Touch Massage

While children, as well as adults, enjoy Light Touch Massage, it should not be used with infants as their nervous system is not developed sufficiently to be able to experience the kind of stimulation that Light Tough offers. After three or four months, you can use Light Touch to calm a fretful child.

TECHNIQUE

The birth companion places the BACK side of his or her fingers so that they meet at the base of the tailbone. The fingers are then drawn up and out from the spine in a V-like motion. The pattern is gradually continued upward across the back until the base of the neck is reached. The hands are then brought around the neck and to the sides of the ears. The undersides of the arms and around the elbows are particularly effective areas for the massage.

The second motion involves placing the BACK of the fingers at the base of the spine and then, as before, gradually working upward, forming a horizontal, figure-eight pattern that crisscrosses at the centre of the back.

This technique will be demonstrated in class, and you will have the opportunity to practise it as well. It is an extremely important element in HypnoBirthing. When the birth companion does it right, the mother will be amazed at the results.

ANCHORS

In the practice of hypnosis, an anchor is a means of creating a lasting imprint or signal through an association with a gesture, sound, image or touch. The thought or suggestion is said to be anchored into the memory of the subconscious. In HypnoBirthing, the birth companion will plant an anchor that is a signal to you to go more deeply into relaxation by placing his hand on your shoulder during your practise sessions. The birth companion instructs the mum that when she feels the hand being placed on her shoulder, with a gentle downward press, she will immediately relax twice as deeply as she is at the moment. You will be amazed at the power of this technique. I suggest that you make it a regular part of your practise together.

Anchors can be used in any number of ways for birthing and in other situations. One woman in a HypnoBirthing class kept forgetting to take her vitamins. She anchored a reminder that when she picked up her car keys to leave in the morning, she would remember to take her vitamins. She never missed a day after that.

Visualisation Techniques

The breathing and relaxation exercises in the previous chapters are fundamental elements of HypnoBirthing and should be practised daily. The visualisation exercises are merely tools to help you during labour. You may find one or all of them useful to calm your mind and relax your body. Therefore, you should experiment to find the ones you like. These visualisation exercises, while helpful, do not need to be part of your daily routine. The exception is Rainbow Relaxation.

RAINBOW RELAXATION

Rainbow Relaxation is the basic visualisation technique of Hypno-Birthing. Mum should practise the entire Rainbow every day by mentally following the outline that follows or with the Rainbow Relaxation CD (available through the HypnoBirthing Institute). If you are in a HypnoBirthing class, your practitioner will provide you with the CD.

The background music, "The Comfort Zone", is a composition by Steven Halpern, a world-renowned author, composer and recording artist whose sounds are designed to bring your thoughts into harmony with the natural flow of energy within your body. We have been using this piece, except for a very brief period of time, since the inception of HypnoBirthing. When we compared the results of the period when we weren't using this tape with the results that we had before and after, we found that there is, indeed, a difference in the ease with which our mothers give birth when using this particular music tape or CD. We enthusiastically suggest that this music is conducive to bringing a labouring mother into a beautifully relaxed and comfortable state, creating a calm and peaceful birthing environment.

You should listen to the entire HypnoBirthing Rainbow Relaxation CD or mentally follow the outline for your own individual practise daily. If there are any words or images on the tape that you don't feel comfortable with, just mentally substitute a word or a phrase that you feel better suits you and let that substitution bring you even deeper into relaxation. All hypnosis is self-hypnosis, and it's important to know that no one else brings you into this state except yourself. Hypnosis is a therapy of consent. If you are finding that you need help in reaching a deep level of relaxation, speak to your practitioner so that together you can get to the root of why this is happening.

Often mums will question if the time they are spending in practise is working for them. They find that after one or two practise sessions, they no longer are able to stay with the material because they drift off into their own thoughts or they fall into a deep sleep. Actually, nothing could be better. If this should happen to you, be aware that you are not actually asleep. You have successfully conditioned your mind to respond immediately by bringing yourself into a state that seems like sleep. If this happens regularly, just know that your subconscious is tuned in to your practise sessions and is processing them for you. That is part of the conditioning effect.

For the purpose of conditioning your mind to relax, Rainbow Relaxation does not have a sequence or "story" to it. The repetition of the wording is especially designed to help you tune out your surroundings and bring you to the level of relaxation that you want to reach quickly. As pleasant as it may be, visualising scenes in nature or spending an inordinate amount of time in progressive relaxation during your practise sessions is not necessary. Whether you mentally visualise the process, your birthing companion walks you through it or you listen to the CD, you will easily master the art after the first week if you allow yourself to just go with it. If you are enjoying the process, you may obtain other discs from the Institute, but the Rainbow exercise will do the trick for you if you are conditioning your mind and body to respond with deep relaxation.

The birth companion is an active participant throughout the birthing experience. Rather than an onlooker who vacillates between feeling helpless and unknowledgeable, in HypnoBirthing the birth companion is actually the trained facilitator and primary support person for the birthing mother. The perinatal bonding that takes place among mother, baby and the birthing companion during this wonderful interlude, combined with the mother's conditioned relaxation, is the whole key to achieving a satisfying birth for all of you.

As often as possible, the birthing companion should practise the Rainbow Relaxation with you, following the outline below. This practise is important so that you will be able to drift into a deep level of relaxation on hearing your birth companion's voice. When you practise with your birth companion, it is better to keep your sessions shorter, but more frequent. This will prevent your time together from becoming a lengthy chore that can be put off until you "can find more time".

While reciting the sequence of colours, the birth companion should stroke your hand and arm in a soft upward motion, simulating the flow of natural relaxation that will drift throughout your body while you are in the thinning and opening phase of labour.

The Birth Companion's Reading (page 110) provides a visualisation of moving through labour that can help you to envision a smooth, calm birth. This can be practised alternately with the Rainbow Relaxation. When you choose to use the Birth Companion's Reading, have the mum picture herself stepping into the happy scene of both of you holding and bonding with your baby seconds after birth. This is an important visualisation for creating an imprint of a positive, happy outcome.

The practise that you do together is intended to strengthen the conditioning that comes from your learning to respond to your birth companion's voice and touch. It will also strengthen the bond between you as you anticipate your upcoming birthing.

TECHNIQUE

- Find a place where you both can be comfortable and where the lighting is soft. Mum should be sitting in a chair with her head resting on the back of the chair or on a sofa with pillows beneath her head and shoulders so that the top of her body is elevated slightly.
- Mum, gently bring yourself into a deep state of relaxation –

the kind you have been teaching yourself. Breathe in relaxation and breathe down relaxation throughout your body, using the Sleep Breathing technique.

- Once you have brought yourself into this calm state of relaxation, picture yourself gently resting on a bed of strawberry-coloured mist that is about a foot and a half high. Picture the soft red mist as a mist of natural relaxation flowing through and around your body. Continue to relax until it seems that your body is almost weightless and seems to meld into the mist. Feel the coloured mist caressing your shoulders, midriff, buttocks and legs. Allow yourself to "let go" and feel as though you are floating on the strawberry-coloured mist. Feel the gentle sway. See this soft mist saturating your body as you go deeper into relaxation. Feel your body growing numb, almost as though it were a piece of soft, strawberry-coloured cloth. Allow yourself to feel the mist of deep relaxation permeating your mind and body from the top of your head to your toes. Feel the tingling of relaxation on the soles of your feet. Imagine your own natural mist of relaxation swirling over and around your body – mind and body at peace and tranquil.

- Now picture yourself resting on a bed of pale, orange-coloured mist, while your body becomes even more comfortable. Follow the same visualisation as you did for the soft strawberry colour. Imagine the coloured mist sweeping across your body, starting at the top of your head, caressing your shoulders, chest, arms and legs, and slowly drifting all the way down to your feet. Again, feel the tingling of relaxation on the soles of your feet and know that you are going deeper in relaxation.

- Next picture yourself on a mist of soft yellow, with the coloured mist surrounding your body, starting at the very top of your head and drifting down across your cheeks, jaws and mouth. Now the same quality of relaxation slips down across your shoulders, upper arms, elbows and hands, and wanders down through your abdomen, legs and to the very bottom of the soles of your feet.

- Continue the visualisation until all the remaining colours of the rainbow have been envisioned – green, blue, indigo, then white for clarity.

- Now slowly bring yourself back to the room, feeling alert and
energised.

Each visualisation will cause you to become more profoundly
relaxed. You may even experience a swaying sensation. This technique and imagery is important as it will be used by the birth
companion along with the Glove Relaxation technique (page 115)
during your birthing. These are the kinds of suggestions that will
facilitate the flow of natural relaxation throughout your body while
you are in the thinning and opening phase of labour.

THE BIRTH COMPANION'S READING

This reading is adapted from one originally composed by Henry Leo
Bolduc for his wife, Joan, when they were preparing for the birth of
their baby. The script appears in Henry's book, *Self-Hypnosis:
Creating Your Own Destiny.*

When I first read Henry's script, I was touched by the beauty of
his words. It is an outpouring of the awe with which a father views
this wonderful miracle. Henry expresses a sensitivity to perinatal
bonding when he points out that the attitude and philosophy of the
mother and the birth companion are as much a gentle suggestion for
the child during birthing as it is reassurance for the mother. Thanks
to Henry for allowing me to incorporate a few HypnoBirthing
images into his script.

New life is forming, growing and moving within you. You are part
of the promise and the destiny of life itself. A very important event
is taking place in your life ... a wonderfully normal, natural, bio-
logical and spiritual event. You're going to have a baby. What is
happening now is the process of birthing and freeing the kicking,
moving little being who's been a part of your body for so long.

Soon it will be time for the baby to become its own separate
person. One cycle is ending and, immediately, another is beginning.
What has been called "labour" is that in-between experience ... the
fulcrum ... that small, short period of time and space between the
baby's two worlds.

Change from one stage to another brings pressure, and then

release. You will soon experience this as the change is completed and fulfilled. You can feel this and embrace it and welcome it as refreshing and totally natural.

With mind, you build a healthy attitude and happy expectation. Happy childbirth has much to do with a healthy, joyous, loving anticipation. It is something remarkably beautiful. Being a channel of new life is said to be a spiritual experience. With this understanding, total relaxation and serene breathing, all discomfort is lessened and often entirely absent.

As you begin labour, meditate on the tremendous universal force ... the life force of nature with which you are in complete harmony during this experience.

Whenever you feel your body begin to surge, actively think "release" and "let go" of tension. There is a time for experiencing that uterine wave, flowing with it, and ultimately releasing and letting go.

You are learning to relax, to flow and melt with the very rhythm of life itself. With relaxation and positive expectation, you have come to know that all things are possible.

In your mind's eye, picture the shore of a lake or an ocean. Watch the endless waves softly brushing to the shore ... the ebb and flow of the water. Observe it advancing and withdrawing over the sand. Become a part of it, flowing into it. Become a part of the rhythm of the waves within your own body ... the surge and release.

Breathe in the natural relaxants of your own body ... endorphins, many times more effective than the strongest drugs known to man ... create your own serenity and release it throughout your body ... breathing in and breathing through ... giving birth to your baby.

With proper physical, spiritual and mental exercise, you are preparing yourself for this wonderful celebration of life. As you get into the rhythm and work with your mind and body, the easier and smoother it becomes. Each time you hear your birth companion's voice and feel the gentle touch, the more easily your relaxation deepens.

Breathe ... slowly, confidently, gently. Each time you breathe in, breathe in relaxation and peace. Each time you breathe out, breathe out stress, as the body's natural endorphins willfully breathe out tension and stress.

Feel only the sway of the wave that is bringing your baby closer and closer to birth. Relax and flow with your body's natural rhythm, confident in the fact that your body knows what to do. Give your birthing over to your body. Trust it. Relax and let it do its job.

With your mind's eye and your inner senses, mentally and emotionally feel yourself joyfully, totally aware and participating. See it as already accomplished. Listen with your mind's ear to that first sound of new life.

Create a vivid visualisation of the exhilaration you feel as you see your baby at the moment of birth. See the three of you bonding for the first time in this life. Now mentally see yourself stepping into this joyful scene. Become a part of this birthing ... fulfilled. Feel it ... sense it. This is your body, here, now. In your mind's eye, see and feel yourself totally enveloping that body ... holding the baby on your breast. These are your arms enfolding your baby; these are your hands embracing this new little being.

You knew you could do it, and you did. You did well, and the feeling of ecstasy is one that will never be surpassed.

Join in with joy and amazement, and watch the continuing mystery of creation unfold. The life force of nature is working in harmony with you. Now more than at any moment in your life, it is within you and with you. You are an integral part of nature, and nature is an integral part of your being. You are a part of the greatest celebration of life.

You are a part of the promise and the destiny of life itself.

THE OPENING BLOSSOM

One of the most simple and effective visualisations is that of an opening rose. Use your breathing techniques to bring yourself into relaxation, then close your eyes and envision your baby moving gently down to the vaginal outlet. Imagine the gradual opening of the perineum to be like the gentle unfolding of the petals of the rose. This visualisation is recommended during the final days of your pregnancy to achieve the onset of labour, and during the opening and birthing phases of labour.

BLUE SATIN RIBBONS

Remember the lower circular muscle fibres that draw up and back to effect the thinning and opening of your cervix? Close your eyes and imagine the muscles, not as fibres, but as soft, blue satin ribbons that gently and easily yield to the rhythmic draw of the vertical muscles, swirling up and back. You can practise this visualisation toward the end of your pregnancy so that it will be there for you during the surges of the thinning and opening phase of your labour.

THE ARM-WRIST RELAXATION TEST

Because you don't really experience a particular sensation when you are in self-hypnosis, you will be amused and amazed at the Arm-Wrist Relaxation Test. It is very simple and, at the same time, very convincing. The technique is meant to assure both the birth companion and the mum that all the practise that you've been doing is working.

TECHNIQUE

Lie on your back, with your arms at your side, your fingers gently cupped on the surface of the bed or sofa. Do not lie flat on your back for long periods of time or when you are in the late stages of pregnancy or in labour.

Once you are in a state of relaxation, picture that your birth companion has tied a giant, helium-filled red balloon to your right wrist. Almost immediately you will feel a tug on your wrist as the balloon pulls upward. Now another helium-filled balloon – this one orange – is added. The two balloons are tugging even harder on your wrist. Your arm is beginning to rise upward. You sense that your elbow is making a dent in the cushion or surface of your bed. The deeper the dent, the more your wrist moves upward. With each tug, your arm is being pulled higher. Still another balloon – a yellow one – is being added. Each time a balloon is added, your arm begins to feel lighter and lighter. The more you try to hold your wrist down, the more the helium is pulling your arm upward. Your arm cannot resist the pull of the balloons. Try as you may to hold it down, your wrist is being yanked upward. Continue to picture more balloons being added with all of the colors of the rainbow.

When your arm rises approximately six to ten inches off the bed, place it back at your side. Each time you practise this exercise, fewer balloons will be required to make your arm and wrist tilt upward. At the end of each relaxation period, tell yourself that each time you practise, relaxation will take over your body sooner than ever before. Your goal should be to assume a deep level of relaxation within a very short period of time.

Ultra-Deepening Techniques

These techniques have been found to be extremely effective in deepening relaxation to a point where the mother's body is totally limp, and she is in an almost amnesiac state. The expanded sessions of these exercises that you will practise in class with your practitioner will help you achieve the deep level of relaxation that you will use during the time that you are nearing completion and beginning to use gentle birth breathing. This total relaxation allows the mum to go within to her birthing body and her baby. Often a mother will remain in this deep state while she breathes her baby down the birth path to the time for the baby to emerge.

To practise this combination of techniques, just breathe yourself into a state of relaxation. Once your body feels comfortably limp, you are ready to proceed.

GLOVE RELAXATION

Glove Relaxation is the first of a combination of deepening techniques, and it is one of the best ways for you and your birth companion to plant an anchor for deep, soothing relaxation. It is also quite effective as a directive during labour and birthing. For this reason, I recommend that it be one of the primary elements of your practise sessions.

TECHNIQUE

Imagine that you are putting a soft, silver glove onto your right hand – a special glove of natural endorphins. Immediately the fingers of your hand begin to feel larger and to tingle, as though there were springs at the ends of your fingers. The silver glove, with its endorphins flowing around your fingers, your palm and the back of your hand, will cause your hand to feel numb, the way it would if you were to place it into a large container of icy slush.

As your birth companion strokes the back of your hand and arm, feel a tingling and then a numbness surrounding your hand and moving up your arm. Once your hand and arm lose all sensation, they begin to seem as lifeless and senseless as a piece of wood or a piece of leather. The silver mist of endorphins gradually drifts throughout your hand so that it can be transferred wherever you wish to bring about relaxation and comfort. To transfer the numbing effect, just visualise placing your hand on various parts of your body – each part now feels light, numb and senseless. Even mums who claim to feel uncomfortable when being touched fall into relaxation when the birth companion uses this technique and recites birthing prompts.

Practise will condition your body to react with calm when you feel your hand and arm being stroked. Go only with your breathing and your visualisations, not your body. Let your body continue to lie totally limp and senseless.

THE DEPTHOMETER

The purpose of this exercise to have you experience bringing yourself into an ultradeep state of relaxation – the kind you will use during the latter part of the opening phase of labour.

TECHNIQUE

In your mind's eye, see or imagine within your body a large, soft, flexible, inverted thermometer. The bulb of the thermometer is just above your forehead. The flexible tube extends all the way down to your toes. Inside the bulb is a clear fluid of natural relaxation.

There are forty gradations on the thermometer. As you count down from 40 to 39 to 38, and so on, picture the fluid of relaxation gently flowing down from one number to the next, flowing out into your circulatory system and bringing your body into relaxation. To reinforce the concept of relaxation filling every cell, nerve and muscle of your body, visualise more fluid flowing down into the tube of the thermometer. You will feel a deep relaxation gradually saturating your body as the fluid fills the space in the tube.

As you slowly count down, the round numbers – 30, 20, 10 and 0 – will bring you to a new and deeper level of relaxation. By the time you reach the lower teens, you will find yourself in a very deep relaxation. The final ten digits will bring you to the ultradeep relaxation you will use during the latter part of the thinning and opening phase of labour.

When your body is thoroughly relaxed, imagine that you are wearing a long, silver glove of relaxation, with the relaxation moving upward in and around your wrist, your lower arm and now all the way to your elbow. Your arm begins to feel almost as though it were not there. Once you experience this sensation, the relaxation can be transferred to other parts of your body, particularly the lower pelvic area. You can use this visualisation alone or with your birthing companion in practise or during labour.

THE SENSORY GATE VALVE

This is a very simple imagery that, like Glove Relaxation, helps to bring about a loss of sensation in selected parts of your body. The imagery of the control valve can be used for any number of things, such as keeping your blood pressure at a safe and healthy level, maintaining a safe amount of amniotic fluid and controlling your stress level.

TECHNIQUE

Once you have mastered the art of bringing yourself into a deep state of natural relaxation, see or imagine yourself in the centre of the inner mind, the Control Room of the subconscious, where you are sitting in front of a large round valve. The valve controls the messages that are sent from the brain, past the sensory gate in the brain stem to all of the nerves in your body. The indicator on the valve is set to the ON position at twelve o'clock, where it is normally as you go about your daily routine. When the valve is on, you can move normally and feel. If you were to injure yourself, you would experience pain.

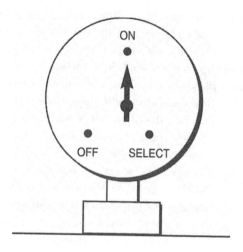

The Sensory Gate Control Valve

To shut off any of those feelings and sensations throughout your body, you can turn the dial to the OFF position at eight o'clock on the dial, and you can feel a sense of well-being begin to sweep over your entire body. Relaxation and comfort begin to set in. You can feel the sensation of relaxation, numbness and tingling begin to be evident in your elbows, knees, lower legs and ankles, then all the way down the soles of your feet. Whenever you feel that tingling at the soles your feet, you know that you are directing the relaxation and endorphins within your body. You can feel sensations of pressure or movement, but you feel a total sense of comfort.

When the dial is in the "Select" position at four o'clock, you can deactivate any part of your body where you choose to experience only comfort and euphoria. Your body becomes conditioned to shut off any message other than that of comfort and relaxation and ease to any given part of your body.

This exercise is helping you to learn how you can practise numbing a hand or any other part of your body, and then transfer that relaxation and numbness to your lower abdomen.

Right now you can move any part of your body, except it now feels as though all sensation has left your right hand. Your hand feels like it is encased in a glove of relaxation. It becomes heavy and numb, almost totally immovable. Your fingers begin to feel larger.

Now you want to transfer the numbness and lack of sensation to the cheek at the right side of your mouth. Feel the numbness now transferring to the right side of your mouth, your tongue, and the tissues in and around the inside of your mouth. Feel that section becoming increasingly numb. Tissues within your mouth begin feeling larger. Now tap the side of your cheek until you have restored the normal feeling throughout that side of your face. Tap until every part of that area is back to normal. Now return your hand to your leg and restore the Glove Relaxation.

Now your hand transfers that heavy numb feeling to your right leg and right foot. The leg and foot are so heavy that it is impossible to move them. Your foot feels as though it is stuck to the floor. Now your right leg on which your hand is resting has become so heavy that it is impossible to lift. Your right foot is so heavy that it seems stuck to the floor. Any attempt now to lift your heavy right leg or lift your foot from the floor is impossible. your foot is stuck. Try to lift your right foot. You cannot.

Now put the indicator back to the normal position of "ON" and return all normal functioning to your entire body. Lift your right hand and right foot. All mobility has returned. Return now to a state of alertness.

With practise you will be able to reach an even deeper level of numbness and relaxation each time. As your labour progresses during birthing, you will find that you are able to go deeper and deeper into this level, transferring the numbness and relaxation to your abdomen and pelvic area with the simulation of the Glove Relaxation. This will help you to keep those areas filled with endorphins and feeling comfortable.

TIME DISTORTION

We know that people who experience hypnosis rarely have a good sense of the length of time that they are in a session. This is a blessing to the birthing mother.

Once you have mastered the art of bringing yourself into relaxation, you may want to begin practising time distortion. When you are in a relaxed state, give yourself the suggestion that every five minutes will seem as one minute. During labour, when you are

nearing the end of your thinning and opening phase, the birth companion will give you the suggestion that every twenty minutes will
seem as five. Time distortion is an important part of birthing and is
included among the prompts used by the birth companion.

   This loss of a sense of time, and the accompanying state of amnesia, comes at a time in labour when you are so deeply relaxed that it
is difficult for you to talk, and you lose a sense of the people around
you. At this time, you will go more deeply into your birthing body
and to your baby, and you will begin your journey together. This is
a gift of nature that can occur with all birthings if the mother is willing to let go, bring herself deep enough and turn her birthing over
to her body and her baby.

> The partner's encouragement and practical help increase the
> effectiveness of labour-coping techniques, such as creative
> imagery and breathing patterns. The presence also increases
> the woman's chance of an emotionally fulfilling birth.
>
> CARL JONES, THE BIRTH PARTNER'S HANDBOOK

Nutrition

We've talked about the emotional, mental and psychological aspects of birthing. These are all important to help you achieve a calm and relaxed birthing. But what you put into your body in the way of nutrition and how you prepare your body physically for birthing can make all the difference in the world in how your birthing plays out. Good nutrition is essential if you hope to have a healthy pregnancy and healthy birth, and intend to sidestep many of the special circumstances of late pregnancy that can turn your birthing around.

WATER: THE MIRACLE LIQUID

Consuming a sufficient amount of water is one of the most important elements in your daily health routine during pregnancy, and it's one of the easiest tasks that you can fit into your schedule. You need to consume water and other liquids, such as juices. to keep your body hydrated for better all-around bodily function. Hydration is paramount.

Approximately 60 per cent of the human body is composed of water. It is one of the chief means of transportation within the body, carrying essential nutrients to the tissues and muscles that need them. Water aids in your digestion by moving food through the digestive system and then moving toxic waste products out of your body in elimination – two very important considerations when you are pregnant. Water acts as a lubricant, as well as a cushion for joints and muscles, and plays a major role in the spinal cord. It also helps to maintain a healthy body temperature. Because pregnancy changes the way your body stores and uses fluids, the kidneys are far more active in filtering toxins. Increasing your consumption of water can aid in this process and help avoid problems with toxemia later in pregnancy.

Water is one of the least expensive ways to maintain good physical health during your pregnancy, and it will help to ensure that you don't experience some of the inconveniences that some pregnant women may encounter, such as joint pain, constipation, muscle cramps, digestive problems and a host of other common annoyances. It is far better to avoid these nuisances than to require steps to treat them.

Water is continually lost through exertion and body heat, as well as through the skin, kidneys, lungs, colon, and urination and perspiration. When you lose water through these means, it needs to be replaced because of the body's need for water. Amniotic fluid is replenished at least three times a day.

You will read and hear many recommendations concerning the amount of water that a pregnant woman should consume. Generally, it is recommended that a pregnant woman drink eight glasses of water daily, or a little over two quarts. You will need to consume more water if your activity level is high, if you live in a higher elevation, if the air where you live is less humid, if air temperatures are high, or if you consume a high-fibre diet, which you may be doing to ward off constipation.

The current thinking in determining how much water you should drink is simple. Allow your body to tell you what it needs, as it so nicely does in many other circumstances. You can easily tell if you are consuming a sufficient amount of water by checking the colour of your urine. A body that is properly hydrated releases urine that is the colour of light lemonade. If your urine is a deeper yellow, you need to reach for water more regularly and increase your consumption of protein. It's that simple.

You will also want to be aware of the quality of water – clean spring water or filtered water is optimal. Being faithful to this regimen can help prevent numerous pregnancy problems, as well as dry skin and other complexion problems.

EATING FOR TWO

No single issue is more important as you carry your baby than the nutrition you provide for him as he develops and grows. Remember, you are building another little person made of bones, organs, tissues, muscles, blood and cells. It doesn't matter how conscientiously you approach any building task and how carefully you think you're building, if the materials that go into the construction are less than the best, your project could prove to be less successful than you would like to see. Building a human being is even more exacting. There is not enough attention paid to nutrition during the birthing year, and next to nothing is focused on nutrition prior to conception, so now is the time to take responsibility for good nutrition for your baby.

The result of glossing over this vital subject is that too many otherwise healthy-appearing women are plagued with problems at the end of their pregnancy. Dr. Tom Brewer refers to these problems in his two books – *Metabolic Toxemia in Late Pregnancy* and *What Every Pregnant Woman Should Know.* We highly recommend that you read these books to learn how to avoid most of the problems that women experience at term.

Since the HypnoBirthing philosophy is also one of avoiding, rather than meeting, the consequences of a poor diet, we have set down a few general suggestions that will help you and your baby to maintain good health. It takes a healthy mother to have a healthy baby. Healthy mothers have fewer low-birthweight infants, fewer incidences of premature birth, fewer cases of PIH (pregnancy-induced hypertension) or simply high blood pressure, and fewer incidences of toxemia. (The last two are generally lumped together, though not accurately, and known as preeclampsia.) In general, the pregnancies and births of healthy mothers are more apt to be "normal". The way to start on the road to good pregnancy health, no matter where you are in your pregnancy, is to realise that you are the single source of nutrition for your baby. If he is going to be well nourished, it's going to have to be through you.

Of course, pregnancy vitamin supplements are fine, but they are just that – supplements – which means that you should consume them in addition to a wholly nutritious diet, not as a substitute for a good food programme. It also means that, like most of the population, when you do your grocery shopping you have to do it defensively. Buy fresh and organic foods as often as possible, rather than processed foods, and become educated as to which fruits and vegetables may have been sprayed with pesticides or treated with preservatives. As with everything in your pregnancy, question. You need to protect your baby.

Note: Though these suggestions have been reviewed by a dietician and have been suggested by nutritionists, if you are experiencing a pregnancy that has special circumstances attached or if you have special food considerations, you will want to consult a nutritionist or dietician rather than follow the course of our suggestions.

The ingredients for growing happy, healthy babies are found in healthful foods. You should plan to increase your daily calorie intake by about 300 calories. Here are a few suggestions:*

Eat:

Lots of protein – 75 to 100 grams a day, taken in several snacks or light meals. Protein is the cornerstone of your nutrition programme. Protein includes such food items as cottage cheese, milk, ice cream, frozen yoghurt, cheeses (except soft cheeses like Camembert, brie and Roquefort), safe fish (see below), peanut butter, lean red meat, poultry, liver, pork, ham, bacon, lamb, veal, tofu, eggs, butter, rabbit, vegetables, nuts and seeds (high sources), and fruits.

Celtic or Mediterranean sea salt with no minerals removed – salt to taste.

Safe fish – increase your intake of safe fish or fish oils, which contain omega-3. Check before buying for possible mercury risks.

Green foods – dark, leafy raw foods, celery, green peppers, apples, broccoli, peas, avocado, string beans, Brussels sprouts, asparagus, lima beans, collard greens, Swiss chard, grapes, limes, beet greens, courgettes, dandelion greens, lettuce, spinach (only occasionally as it can limit the absorption of calcium), watercress, snow peas.

Orange foods – squash, yams and sweet potatoes, cantaloupe,

*Sources include the National Dairy Council, Dr. Thomas Brewer's book *Metabolic Toxemia in Late Pregnancy*, the Blue Ribbon Babies Web site, and miscellaneous articles on nutrition.

oranges, peaches, apricots, nectarines, pumpkin, tangerines, carrots, peppers (raw and cooked).

Red foods – watermelon, strawberries (if not sprayed with pesticides), peppers (raw or cooked), tomatoes, apples, raspberries (drink red raspberry leaf tea), cherries, rhubarb, red potatoes, pimiento, radishes.

Coloured fruits – pineapple, pears, bananas, honeydew melons, kiwi, grapes.

Avoid:
  Alcohol
  Caffeine
  Nicotine
  Processed meats – hot dogs, luncheon meats, bologna, liverwurst.
  Raw fish – oysters, sushi and others.
  Unnecessary fats – fried foods, French fries, fast foods.
  White foods – refined sugar, white flour products, white rice, white potatoes.
  Sweets – candies with empty calories that have no nutritional value.

Exercise

It is particularly important that you exercise during pregnancy. It is also crucial, however, that you don't build exercising into a routine that becomes an ordeal or a time-consuming chore. You will want to find ways to tone your body that are as natural as the birthing you are preparing for. Vary the exercises that you do and create a habit of doing them as often as you can as you go about your day-to-day activities.

You'll discover that many exercises can be practised incidentally. Some can even be done right on your bed as you awaken in the morning or just before you settle in for the night. If you are accustomed to brisk exercise, consult with your care provider to be sure that this kind of exercise will not compromise your baby's well-being.

One of the best ways to ensure that you are exercising regularly is to join a prenatal fitness and exercise group. Most of the time, the mothers in these classes are pretty upbeat about their pregnancies and upcoming birthings. Avoid any group that is given to commiserating over bad birth stories.

WALKING

Walking is one of the best exercises you can do. It helps to strengthen your breathing, as well as your legs. You don't have to follow a strict regimen of walking, but you can look for ways to get in a little extra walking time, for example, by parking a distance from the entrance to your work or from the supermarket. Use an entrance that is not immediately adjacent to your destination. Rather than telephoning or taking an elevator to another area, find occasions to walk within the building at work. Walk as often as you can. Be sure that the surfaces you walk on are smooth and safe, and wear sensible shoes. Brisk walking is good from the beginning to the middle of your pregnancy. After that you may want to slow down a bit so that your baby is not jostled too much. When you engage in brisk exercise, your blood is directed to your arms and legs and away from the uterus, meaning that your baby is perhaps not receiving the amount of oxygenated blood that he should. Temper your time and pace.

AVOID BACK STRAIN: PRACTISE GOOD POSTURE

As your pregnancy advances, you will want to alleviate back strain by being aware of correct posture. Pregnant or not, a good assist to proper posture is to envision a string passing from a point at the front of the earlobe, down through the shoulders and the hipbone to a spot just behind the ankle bone. Keeping your head in line with this imaginary string will prevent you from "leading with your head", keep your pelvis tilted back, and help you to avoid stooping as you gain in weight and size.

Don't lean back with your head behind the imaginary line; it will cause you to project your abdomen forward and will lead to the "pregnancy waddle". Many women assume this posture, with toes turned outward, as depicted in comedy skits and sitcoms, long before final "dropping" has occurred. Even then, awareness of how you carry yourself and your baby can make a difference in how you feel at the end of a day.

One of the best devices for maintaining good posture and for helping to ensure that your baby will assume a favourable position for birthing is to avoid slouching down into your pelvic area. This is not too easy to do with so many cars being equipped with bucket seats today, but it can be remedied by placing a pillow on the seat so that it is more level. Avoiding recliners is also good advice for the pregnant woman who is interested in achieving an optimal position for her baby at birth.

One of the best ways to practise good posture when sitting is to regularly sit on a birth ball (also known as an exercise ball). These handy balls can be bought at any number of locations at very reasonable prices, including most sporting goods stores. The birth ball allows you to sit erect, and at the same time tones your inner thighs and pelvic region. Use it at your desk or as a place to relax at home, instead of a chair. The birth ball comes in handy later in pregnancy, and it is a great place to rock during labour. It is one of the best and simplest tools you can buy.

Another exercise that is helpful in relieving back strain is the "pelvic rock". This exercise helps to avoid back strain, strengthens abdominal muscles, increases the flexibility of your lower back and promotes good alignment in your spine. There are several ways to do the pelvic rock. Instructions for two methods follow.

First Method: Using a sturdy chair or other piece of furniture for arm support and balance, stand approximately two feet from the object. Bend your knees very slightly.

Lean forward from your hips and thrust your buttocks backward. Keep your back straight. Allow your abdominal muscles to relax for a few seconds while you create sway.

Bend your knees a little more and pull your hips forward, tucking your buttocks under as though you were being shooed from behind with a broom. Repeat the procedure several times.

Second Method: You can also practise the pelvic rock or tilt in a lying position during the early months of your pregnancy. Once your baby begins to take on some weight, you will want to avoid lying flat on your back.

On your back with your knees bent and your feet flat on the floor, tighten your lower abdominal muscles and the muscles of your buttocks. Your tailbone will rise, pressing the small of your back to the floor. Hold this position for a few seconds and then release the muscles. As you do this exercise, arch your back as much as you can. Repeat the procedure several times.

You will also find this an excellent technique for flattening the abdomen following birthing.

TONING THE INNER THIGH AND LEG MUSCLES

Toning your inner thighs and legs is vitally important for successful labour. At the end of your birthing when you are breathing your baby down and out of the birth path, you may find yourself in many positions that will call for you to use your legs in ways that are a bit unusual. The muscles in your inner thigh will need to be ready.

Position One: The best effect in toning can be derived from sitting on the floor or in the middle of a bed with the soles of your feet together. Lean slightly forward and place your hands on your ankles. With your elbows resting on the inside of your knees, gently press your elbows onto your knees. Do not apply force as you stretch these important groin muscles. As you do this exercise over time, gradually and gently pull your heels toward your crotch until your heels and your crotch meet and your knees almost rest on the floor. Do not rush to make this happen. Take it slowly. Once you have achieved this muscle tone, you should straighten your back during subsequent practise sessions.

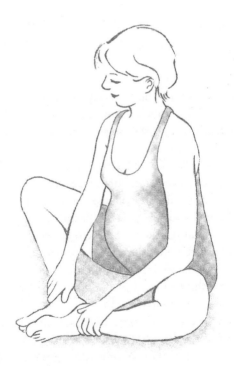

Toning the Inner Thigh Muscles

You can do this exercise alone, but it's more fun to get your birthing companion involved. Using the same technique as described previously, have the birth companion assist from behind you by placing his or her hands under your knees, pressing upward to create resistance. While this is happening, you gently press down on your knees. Then have your birth companion press downward on your knees while you bring your legs upward and push against the pressure.

Position Two: Resting on your tailbone with your knees bent and raised upward toward your shoulders, place the palms of your hands against the inner part of your knees and push your knees outward. Bring your knees together again and then push them apart. Do this about ten times in each practise session.

When you reach for low objects or lift an object or a small child, bend with your knees, rather than from the waist. Do not attempt to lift heavy objects.

THE LEAPING FROG

The Leaping Frog position comes to us from midwives in the Virgin Islands. This easy, forward squat is used in many places in the world. Not only does this position help to tone your muscles, but it also provides you with one of the best positions in which to labour during the birthing phase.

While women in other cultures regularly use a squatting position for birthing, you must remember that these women use this posture for much of what they do on a daily basis. Western women are not naturally inclined to squatting, so this posture needs practise. There are two ways of assuming the Leaping Frog stance – with your arms thrust forward inside your spread knees or with your arms behind you at the side of your hips. The second position is an ideal position to assume for birthing as it relieves all pressure from the buttocks, and provides open and clear access for both baby and attendant. The time that you spend in practising this modified form of squatting will be well spent.

Assuming the Leaping Frog position during labour offers benefits for both you and your baby when you are Birth Breathing. Just a few of the benefits of the Leaping Frog are:

- Widens the pelvic opening
- Relaxes and opens the perineal tissues
- Helps to avoid tearing and lessens the need for an episiotomy
- Relieves strain in the lower back
- Increases the supply of oxygen to your baby
- Shortens the birth path
- Allows you a clear view of your baby's birth
- Makes good use of the effect of gravity

Though I recommend the Leaping Frog position, attempting to adopt it for any length of time when your muscles are not adequately toned could result in pain or injury to your leg muscles. If you choose to birth with your arms behind you, you will want to tone your arm muscles. It's worth spending some time in practise as it is an ideal birthing position.

TECHNIQUE

When first practising the Leaping Frog position, you may need some help in the way of support to get down into the proper position. Your birthing companion can help by standing behind you so that you can lean your back against his legs while he holds your hands for balance. The companion can also stand in front of you to assist as you slowly lower your body into position.

From a standing position with your feet spread about a foot and a half apart, assume a squatting position on your toes with your knees spread outward. Place your hands on the floor on either the inside or the outside of your legs.

A variation of this position is to assume a kneeling position with your legs spread wide and to the side. Lower your body onto your legs, with your buttocks resting on your heels. Place your hands in front of you. This position can be converted into an all-fours stance by simply moving your hands farther front and raising your buttocks as you bring your body forward into a Hands-and-Knees position. This is an excellent position to use for birthing, as well. During birthing, you may wish to place pillows beneath your hands and knees.

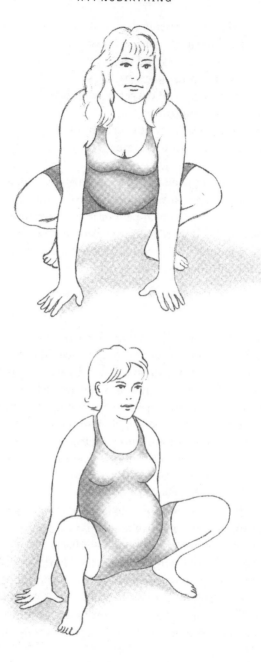

Leaping Frog Positions

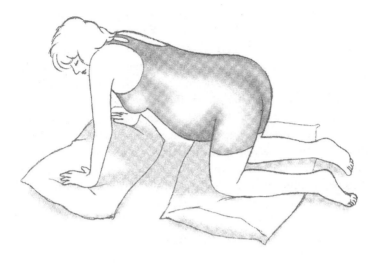

Hands-and-Knees Position for Practise or Birthing

PELVIC FLOOR EXERCISES

Not enough attention is paid to pelvic floor exercises, sometimes called Kegels. They are among the most important of all the pre-natal muscle toning. Designed to tone and strengthen the muscles used during the birthing phase of labour, these exercises involve the network of muscles that form a figure eight around the entire vaginal and anal region.

Toning the pelvic floor muscles also serves the very important function of quick return to their normal size after labour and can be helpful in preventing some of the urinary problems connected with aging. Control of this area can actually enhance lovemaking after having a child. You will enjoy the confidence derived from well-toned anal and vaginal sphincters as your pregnancy advances and there is more pressure on the bladder and bowel.

TECHNIQUE

In a sitting position, start by contracting the lowest muscles of the anal and vaginal tracts as tightly as you can. Keep tightening the vaginal muscles until you can feel the contracted muscles all the way up into the top of the vagina. When working with anal muscles, draw in until you get the sensation of pulling the anus into the rectum. It is helpful, though not necessary, to count from one to ten as you do these exercises, tightening a little more with each number. When you have tightened the muscles in the area, hold the contraction for a few seconds and then release slowly.

These muscles are the same ones used to stop the flow of urine. To see if you are doing this exercise correctly, attempt to stop the flow of urine while you are urinating. Do not continue to do this once you have established that you are doing the exercise correctly. To do this more than is necessary could result in a urinary tract infection. Be sure to practise this exercise several times a day, doing the exercise five to ten times at each practise. Frequent practise is all to your benefit. These exercises can be done easily at any time, anywhere, whether at work or at home, while driving or while walking. The important thing is to DO IT.

Perineal Massage

Perineal massage is one of the oldest and surest ways of improving the health, blood flow, elasticity and relaxation of the pelvic floor muscles. Practised in the latter part of your pregnancy, approximately six to eight weeks prior to term, this technique will also help you to identify and become acquainted with the tissues you will relax and the region through which you will birth your baby. *Perineal massage is vitally important to the success of your HypnoBirth.* Do not take this exercise for granted.

Massaging with oil helps the perineal tissues to soften and thereby gently unfold with no resistance as they open during birthing to allow the passage of the baby. As you or your partner do the massage, you can teach these muscles to relax and open outward in response to pressure.

This massage increases your chances of birthing your baby over an intact perineum. When your perineal rim is soft and relaxed, your baby easily slips past the rim and out of the vagina. Attention to this massage will pay off. It is simple, yet so effective. You will want to take it seriously. The massage should be done *every day for at least five minutes.*

Because of your increased size and the awkwardness of bending around your abdomen, it may be easier to have someone else do the massage for you. If the massage is done gently, there is no need for discomfort. I suggest that couples make it part of their lovemaking.

If you are doing the massage by yourself, you'll find it easier if you place one foot on the seat of a chair, with the other approximately two or three feet away from the chair. This allows you to work around and under your abdomen from the back.

Be sure that fingernails are smooth and short when doing the massage. A rubber glove will ensure that there are no rough surfaces to irritate the vaginal tissue. You may use virgin olive oil, sweet oil, almond oil, apricot oil or a lubricating gel. Avoid perfumed oils.

TECHNIQUE

Pour a little of the oil into an egg cup or shallow bowl. (Be sure to discard oil that is left after massaging – do not reuse.)

Sit with your back resting against pillows and get comfortable. It's a good idea to use a mirror during the first few times that you do this exercise. It will assist you in identifying the muscles involved and allow you to observe the easing of the edge of the perineum.

Dip your thumb into the oil and thoroughly moisten it. If a partner is doing the massage, he will use his first and middle fingers. The thumb or fingers should be dipped into the oil to the second knuckle and inserted into the vagina approximately two to three inches, pressing downward on the area between the vagina and the rectum. Rub the oil into the inner edge of the perineum and the lower vaginal wall.

Maintaining a steady pressure, slide the fingers upward along the sides of the vagina in a U, sling-type motion. This pressure will stretch the vaginal tissue, the muscles surrounding the vagina and the outer rim of the perineum. Be sure to stretch the inner portions as well as the outer rim of the perineum. In the beginning you will feel the tightness of the muscles, but with time and practise, the tissue will relax.

Practise relaxing the extended muscles by picturing the perineum opening outward as pressure is applied. The opening rosebud is a good visualisation to use during this exercise.

Getting Ready to Welcome Your Baby

Do be positive. Convey two messages:
First, this is a well-researched baby, and you are a prepared
and informed parent. You are doing everything you can do
to take care of your health and the health of your baby.
Second, you are asking your caregivers to do likewise.

WILLIAM SEARS AND MARTHA SEARS, *THE BIRTH BOOK*

So far you've been doing all of the right things in preparing yourself
mentally, emotionally and physically for your baby's birth. Now it's
time to start tying the ends together.

If you and your birth companion have a clear vision of what will
allow you to have the most natural, gentle and satisfying birth experience for you and your baby, you won't find yourselves looking
on as your birthing is controlled by others.

The best way to ensure that your birth experience is positive,
healthy and safe for you and your baby is to thoroughly prepare and
plan. Sitting down together and deciding what is important to you
and safe for your baby will certainly increase your chances of being
able to experience the most satisfying birth. In the absence of Birth
Preference Sheets, hospital staff and birth attendants cannot know
what you are looking for in your birthing experience.

YOUR BIRTH PREFERENCES

Too often couples come away from their birthing experiences
expressing their disappointment with phrases such as, "Oh well,
the next time ..." or, "If only they hadn't ..."

Now is the time to get specific. Hopefully, you have secured the right caregiver who listens to you and respects your wishes. This can add to your confidence that your birthing will not needlessly turn into a "medical incident". You cannot assume, though, that because you talked with your caregiver at the onset of your pregnancy, he or she will remember your conversation when it comes time to birth. That's what Birth Preference Sheets are about. Talking with your doctor or midwife about your birth preferences should take place early and often in your pregnancy and not simply left to a chance conversation as you approach term. You will still have to remind the caregiver that together you agreed that this is to be a natural birth if at all possible. If you did your homework as you made your selection of a caregiver and a birthing environment, this shouldn't be a problem.

Bring additional copies with you to each antenatal visit so that you can speak with each of the people who will possibly attend your birth. If you plan to have a homebirth or to birth in a birthing centre, you will want to see that your midwife, and anyone else who will be present, has a copy.

Any guests who are planning to attend your birth should know that you have a plan in place and that your birthing is not the time for them to relate stories of the progress of their own labours or in any way attempt to influence the course of your labour by giving advice. Because it can be awkward for you and your birth companion if conflict should arise, it is a good idea to have anyone who will be at your birthing attend HypnoBirthing classes with you. If this is impossible, the matter should definitely be discussed prior to the time of labour. It is important that everyone at the birth understand what you are doing and that they have a sense of your need for a calm and restful environment.

You might want to think twice about inviting people other than a professional labour companion into your labour. When you think back to the ambiance of the lovemaking that resulted in your conceiving this baby, consider having that same ambiance at birth – the dimly lit room, privacy, music, no interruptions. This is the atmosphere that should surround the birth of your child.

A veteran labour and birthing nurse once told me, half seriously, that the number of people in the birthing room beyond the couple and their labour companion seemed to extend the labour by an hour for each person. You want only good birthing energy in your labour room. You are the stars, directors and producers in this play. You call the shots.

In presenting your birth preferences to your health-care providers, keep in mind that your intent is not to "take on" your medical caregivers or practices that are currently in effect in the hospital or centre. The HypnoBirthing Birth Preference Sheets are worded in such a way that they do not take on the aura of an adversarial document of demands. When you discuss your birth preferences, you will also want to assure your medical providers that they will have your full co-operation should a medical necessity arise.

A suggested outline for your birth preferences appears at the end of this book. Your HypnoBirthing instructor will give you a worksheet for your own use, along with a letter to your health-care provider. Depending on where you live, some of the choices on your preferences may already be "standard" for that facility. You should inquire about that when you broach the subject of preferences during your tour. You may skip any items that you do not feel strongly about or write N/A in front of those that you know are already in effect. There is room on the plan after each section to put additional requests or comments.

So what's important on the Birth Preference Sheets? According to Dr. Lorne Campbell, "It's all important, and each item that you care about needs to be addressed". Parents need to repeat their wishes clearly throughout pregnancy and when they are admitted to their birthing facility.

If you hear that midwives don't read Birth Preference Sheets, and that they see them as a map that leads directly to the operating room, you have to remember that is a bias that is no longer true in most places. Our Birth Preference Sheets are respectful and do not ask for anything that would require exceptional effort. Just the opposite is true. The preferences request less than what is routine. Because some staff may prefer a one-page Birth Preference Sheet is no reason to compromise the other items in the plan. Condensing it is not going to honour your wishes.

When you are admitted at the hospital for your birthing, ask your midwife to take a few minutes with you to go over your Birth Preference Sheets. You may need to make that request again as shifts change and provide the new midwife on duty with a copy of your birth preferences. In some hospitals where HypnoBirthing has been in place for several years, the midwives initiate the discussion of your birth preferences and will sit down with the couples after they have been admitted to go over them.

HOSPITAL OR BIRTHING CENTRE VISIT

HypnoBirthing provides you with information and techniques that help you develop confidence as you approach your birthing. To add another measure of confidence, it is helpful for you and your birthing companion to visit the hospital or birthing centre again sometime in advance of your anticipated birthing. Getting these "housekeeping duties" out of the way will ensure that you will not get bogged down with unnecessary delays at the time of your admission. Take advantage of the opportunity to talk with staff and complete paperwork. It's a good idea to call ahead to be sure that you are not planning to show up on a day when every room is filled with mums having babies. Ask for a nurse who is partial to natural birthing for your tour guide; otherwise, you may get more than you want to see and hear.

Inform the staff that you are planning a relaxed birthing with HypnoBirthing and that it be noted in your file. Be sure to leave a copy of your Birth Preference Sheets and request that it be added to your records. If this is a first HypnoBirthing at this facility, take the time to explain a little about the method and ask about the things they do to accommodate natural birth. If the facility has a birthing tub, they will welcome the opportunity to show it off. Even if you are not planning to birth in water, this is a good time to discuss gentle birth.

Use this visit to become familiar with the layout and environment of the centre. Inquire about entrances that should be used in the event you arrive before or after the hours that the hospital or centre is normally open to the public. Know where lifts and reception desks are located. You don't want to find yourselves wandering around lost at a time when you should be "settling in" to your birthing.

It's helpful to have an idea of the time it takes to travel to the centre. Do a couple of "dry runs" – one during a heavily trafficked time of day and one on a Sunday or late evening. Check out alternative routes that may not be as heavily travelled as the one you usually take.

When Baby is Breech

In preparation for birthing, sometime between the thirty-second and thirty-seventh weeks of pregnancy, the baby turns from its upright position into what is called a *vertex position* in preparation for birthing. With this turn, the baby's head is properly positioned down at the mouth of the cervix. Because the head contains the brain and the skull, it is the heaviest part of the baby's body. Once the baby is almost fully developed, the natural pull of gravity is usually sufficient to draw the head down.

Most of the time this turning goes without note, especially if it occurs while the mum is sleeping. The turn can be delayed, however, if the mum is experiencing fear or tension, or if there are circumstances in her life that are upsetting.

Some mums, for any number of reasons, are reluctant to "let go", and so their uterus remains taut and the baby is not able to complete the turn. When this happens, the baby, deprived of adequate space in which to turn, is unable to complete the rotation and remains in the original, upright position. The baby's buttocks remain at the neck of the uterus in what is called "breech presentation". Sometimes the baby completes only a partial rotation, leaving a shoulder, an arm, or one or both feet positioned at the lower part of the cervix.

A breech position, if not reversed, calls for important decisions. The options are limited to making every effort to help the baby turn, to birth the baby in the breech position, or to resort to a surgical birth. Since few medical providers are trained in the birthing of breech-presented babies, most resort to caesarean births, but this doesn't need to be the first avenue to explore. Many women birth their breech-presented babies vaginally with homebirth midwives.

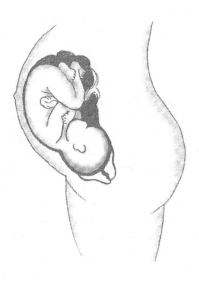

Proper Vertex Position

HELPING THE BREECH-POSITIONED BABY TO TURN

Many babies have been coached to turn with the help of HypnoBirthing techniques. A special session has proven to be very effective in helping the breech-presented baby to spontaneously reposition into vertex position on its own. This concept is buttressed in a study, presented by Dr. Lewis Mehl-Madronna, formerly of the psychiatric department of the University of Vermont Medical School and Arizona University School of Medicine. The study included 100 women who were referred from practicing obstetricians and an additional 100 who responded to an advertisement. Only women who were found to be carrying their babies in breech position at thirty-six weeks gestation or more were included. Mehl-Madronna approached this study looking at reports on serial ultrasound examinations and abdominal palpation that suggested that the likelihood of a breech-positioned baby turning after the thirty-seventh week was no more than 12 per cent.

One hundred women in the study group used hypnotherapy.

The comparison group of 100 women had no hypnotherapy, though some did have ECV (external cephalic version), a procedure whereby the baby's head is manually manipulated from outside the abdomen to bring about the downward turn.

In the study group, the mothers, while in hypnosis, were led through guided imagery to bring about deep relaxation. Suggestions were then given that they visualise their babies easily turning and see the turn accomplished, with the baby in proper vertex position for birthing. The mothers were helped to visualise the uterus becoming pliable and relaxed in order to allow the baby sufficient room to make the move. The mother was asked to talk to her baby, and the therapists encouraged the baby to release itself from the position it had settled into and to turn downward for an easy birth.

The study ended with 81 of the 100 breech babies in the study group having turned spontaneously from breech position to vertex position. It was originally thought that each mother would require approximately ten hours of hypnotherapy in order to accomplish the desired result. As the study unfolded, the average number of hours spent with each woman was only four, and half of the successful 81 turns required only one session.

In the comparison group of 100 women who did not participate in hypnotherapy, only twenty-six babies turned spontaneously. An additional twenty were turned with ECV. It should be noted that it is not uncommon for the baby who is turned through ECV to turn back into breech position. The figures arrived at through this study are considered medically quite significant.

From these findings we see that, in addition to working with visualisation conducive to relaxing the uterus, mothers with babies in breech position can be helped through release therapy. Release therapy is an integral part of the HypnoBirthing programme, where mothers are helped to identify and release negative emotions. If your baby is in breech presentation and there is talk of a possible surgical birth, seek the assistance of your HypnoBirthing practitioner, who will help you with a special hypnosis session that has been found to be especially successful in achieving the desired turn. When the turning of the breech baby is achieved through relaxation and tension release, the baby usually remains in vertex position.

Your practitioner can also help you with finding community resources, acupuncturists, acupressurists and chiropractors who perform the Webster technique, reflexologists and others who can help with turning techniques. Inquire about "tilting" techniques and other methods for helping the baby to turn. Then, and only then, consider ECV if it is still necessary. ECV should be a last resort. It is not usually a procedure of choice for most women, but it is preferable to surrendering to a surgical birth.

Before Labour:
When Baby Is Ready

From working with HypnoBirthing mothers over many years, I find that our mothers welcome the early signs that labour is near. Sometime prior to term, the mother begins to sense various signals that nature is playing its part in tuning up for the main concert.

EARLY SIGNALS

Practise Labour: Much talked about, but little understood, these surges are nature's way of preparing the uterus for your baby's birthing. They are much like the tightening sensations that are felt during labour, and for that reason we call them practise labour. For first babies, these tightening surges will probably show up sometime during the end of the seventh month. For subsequent pregnancies, they may appear as early as the sixth month.

From day-to-day you'll experience more of the practise labour surges. As you move and walk, you may even feel a sharp jolt as the pelvic area begins to make room for the baby's journey. This is the pubis bone moving forward and pulling at a ligament here or there. Your body is telling you that it, too, is "getting ready".

Until the final month of pregnancy, these surges are usually erratic and infrequent. As you come near to term, however, you may find that the intervals between them become shorter, and then finally become as frequent as ten- to twenty-minute intervals. Interestingly enough, these surges will sometimes give you a jolt with their pressure-like waves, but they are not accompanied by pain. This makes one wonder if the painless pre-labour sensations are further proof of the mind-body connection – the mind knows the body is not ready for labour, so no pain impulse is emitted.

While most people don't consider these surges to be labour, there are many who would disagree and support the belief that the body is already involved in a labour practise that does, in fact, result in the cervix beginning to open. Some mums will welcome the opportunity to remain relaxed and greet the surges with ease. As you reach term, you will want to take more notice of these sensations so that you don't dismiss what could actually be labour. Many mums at this time get tuned in to their bodies, and they depend upon this and their instincts to let them know when the real thing has arrived.

Lightening: Several weeks before actual labour begins, the baby "drops" into the lower pelvic area. This is called "lightening". This is usually accompanied by mixed reactions on the part of the mother. It does, indeed, relieve that cramped feeling under the rib cage, and breathing is much easier. However, it also brings about much more pressure on the lower pelvis, and walking becomes a whole new experience. In spite of adjustments that you will have to make for this new position of your baby, you will find, like most other mothers, that your excitement begins to build.

Vaginal Discharge: Occasionally, you may experience more than a slight vaginal discharge that can be clear or whitish. This is another signal that your body is preparing for birth, and it is due to a higher volume of blood flow to that region of your body – another signal that your body is preparing for birth.

LOOKING AT YOUR "DUE DATE"

What if your Estimated Due Date (EDD) arrives and labour does not start? A whole new set of feelings can spring up. Emotionally and physically, you feel ready "to go" – to birth your baby – but it isn't happening. If you take your due date as gospel and you're not prepared for a possible delay, these days of anticipation can take a toll on you. You may find that anxious, well-meaning family members begin to call regularly to check; your doctor will begin to take a more watchful eye; fears concerning the baby's well-being can creep in; and each day can start and end with a feeling of disappointment.

Perhaps you'll hear many stories from your friends who chose to be induced when the baby was "overdue". You may even be tempted to accept the subtle suggestions that you don't really need to wait any longer or that "you can be home for the holiday or the weekend". The important thing for you to do is to continue to relax and wait. Your baby knows when it's time to be born. Trust him or her.

Before overreacting to outside pressures, remember that the estimated due date is just that – an estimation. One of our doctors calls it "The Guess Date". Some suggest that it would be more realistic to refer to a birth month or to a segment of the month – "toward the end of September ..." or "Sometime during the first part of October ..."

There are several reasons why your due date is only an estimation. To begin with, the selected date is usually calculated by recalling the date of the first day of your last menstrual period (which may not be accurate), counting back three months from that date and then adding seven days. However, recent studies suggest that for first-time mums, fifteen days should be added, and ten days should be added for mums who have birthed previously.

There are several factors that can skew this estimate: a) Actual calendar months differ in length; b) Menstrual cycles differ in the number of days between periods and in the duration of a period; c) The length of gestation can vary; d) Detection of a heartbeat or foetal movement may seem to support the timely development of the baby at a given point, but it must be remembered that just as children differ in their development, so, too, do babies in utero.

It's interesting to note that the number of babies who arrive on their due date is only around 5 per cent, so if your birthing is not "on time" relax. You will be among the 95 per cent of parents whose babies are born in advance of the EDD or sometime after the appointed date. The gestation period for 95 per cent of normal babies lies within a very broad range of 265 to 300 days from the first day of the mother's last period. The average, taken from those figures, is the 282 days usually used to estimate the due date.

Also interesting is the fact that so many women today are being given as many as three different "due dates" as they proceed through pregnancy. That is certainly an indication that estimates are not solid. How many times did your conception date change?

You need to be able to focus on the fact that the range is between thirty-eight and forty-two weeks. You are not actually "Post Date" until you reach forty-two weeks. Many physicians will not even consider artificial initiation of labour in the absence of any special circumstances until you are at forty-two weeks. Your EDD has no magical significance, and as long as your baby is strong and healthy and you are strong and healthy, don't allow yourself to be pressured into thinking that every day beyond the EDD is a precarious time.

For your baby's sake, resist the temptation to bring medical intervention to your pregnancy when you pass your Guess Date, and certainly don't even consider induction prior to the EDD without a valid medical indication. Induction should occur only when a medical necessity exists for you or your baby. The artificial induction of labour for a baby whose term has been mistakenly calculated could result in birthing a premature baby. It can also mean further medical procedures if your cervix is not "ripe" and ready for birthing.

If it is suggested that you be induced, you owe it to yourself and your baby to have a valid explanation of the reason. You will want to ask about the risks of induction at the time it is recommended, as well as the benefits. Ask to know what your rating is on the "Bishop's Score", which is used to determine the degree to which your body is ready for labour and the probable success of your being induced. Inductions with low Bishop's Scores could mean that the induction could be difficult, leading to lengthy, painful labour and an increased possibility of surgical birth. A score of 8 or 9 would indicate that the induction probably would be successful, but it could also indicate that your baby's birth is near. An induction should be considered only if there is some true medical indication for it.

If you've done a good job initially at securing the support of your caregiver, this should not become a problem for you.

A chart of the Bishop's Score, showing the categories that are considered, follows.

Cervix	Score			
	0	1	2	3
Position	Posterior	Midposition	Anterior	Anterior
Consistency	Firm	Medium	Soft	Soft
Effacement	0–30%	40–50%	60–70%	80+
Dilation	Closed	1–2 cms	3–4cms	5 cms+
Station	–3	–2	–1	+1,+2

BISHOP'S SCORE CHART

Neither your body nor your baby understands arbitrary time-tables or charts, so take the due date in stride and let Mother Nature and your baby play out their intended roles in their own time. It is the safest and most natural way. Once intervention is introduced in the way of artificial induction, you have already moved away from normal birth. Even the casual suggestion of "just popping that bag" or "doing a little sweep" can change the whole ball game for your birthing.

The best advice in looking at your due date is "don't".

Letting Your Baby
and Your Body Set the Pace

The actual trigger for the beginning of labour is not entirely known, but it is believed that a hormone secreted from within the baby's body triggers oxytocin, the natural labour-initiating hormone within the mother's body, and the miracle unfolds. That is all part of the master plan – a plan that has a designated flow, but not a designated schedule.

A labour that is slow to start or, later, a resting labour, does not automatically call for the introduction of a chemical stimulant to start or speed up your labour. Nor do these indications necessarily mean a complicated labour. If you experience a latent period when your surges are not starting, or if later the distance between the surges is lengthening, it doesn't mean that your birthing has gone askew. It simply means that the uterus and your baby are not so sure that this is the time yet.

Discussion of rushing in to "jumpstart labour" or "move things along" or "augment sluggish surges" can actually bring about the opposite effect and cause a total interruption of the kind of labour that you are planning. If such a comment is made, you or your birthing companion can nicely explain that unless there is a medical urgency, you would like to stay with your birth preferences and that you are in no hurry. One father, when told that if they didn't agree to inducing labour, they could be there all day, commented, "Oh, that's okay. We're not going anywhere." Nature will have its way, and calm is what you need.

Occasionally, a mum will find that even when she accepts the suggestion of rupturing her membranes or of using a vaginal gel or Syntocinon drip, her labour still does not move along. Perhaps her body is being prompted into a labour for which it is not quite ready.

Since the development of brain cells is accelerated during the last eight weeks of pregnancy, it seems prudent to let the baby complete this development in utero and not rush birth.

Once artificial induction or augmentation has been introduced in any form, you may find that you have surrendered your choices. Before agreeing to the introduction of procedures or drugs into your body and, therefore, your baby's body, weigh the possibility that you may be placing yourself and your baby on a very slippery slope.

Some women find that with small doses of synthetic oxytocin, they are able to continue to call on their HypnoBirthing relaxation techniques; others tell us that they tried, but, eventually, Syntocinon won out. They had to request an epidural. This is one of the best reasons for not agreeing to it in the first place unless there is a true medical indication to consider. And, again, we turn to the argument for hiring the right caregiver. When the family and caregiver are working together, this discussion will be moot. You will trust that such recommendations will be given only in the event of a change in the course of your pregnancy or labour that genuinely needs to be remedied by medical assistance.

Few expectant parents really take the time beforehand to explore the risks of deciding to use drugs for faster birth. Parents rarely seek an opportunity to talk with their caregivers about the effects of narcotics upon their pre-born, and subsequently, newborn. No parent would ever choose to give drugs to his or her newborn baby needlessly, but fear of labour can be strong enough to make it simpler for the pregnant family to avoid questions concerning the risks of inductions or epidurals. Similarly, few doctors take the opportunity to explain the adverse side effects of labour drugs with their patients. The matter becomes the medical version of "Don't ask; don't tell".

The well-respected *Physicians' Desk Reference (PDR)* clearly states that at this time there are no adequate and well-controlled studies for the use of these drugs with pregnant women. The *PDR* also points out that it is still not known whether these drugs can cause foetal harm when administered to labouring women. There is no hard evidence to support most of these procedures.

Even pills, or any of the injected drugs used to "take the edge off", can suppress a labouring mum's efforts to work with her body's surges, as HypnoBirthing mums are trained to do. An epidural, used to quell the effects of Syntocinon, may offer relief, but it also has a downside. These narcotics can cause reduced muscle tone and prolong labour. Because of the numbing effects of drugs, the labouring woman is less aware of her surges and may not be able to efficiently assist in working with them to facilitate opening. This can prolong labour and often results in increased administration of Syntocinon, leading to continued pain relievers, and so on. A very vicious cycle is established. If she is unable to feel surges and assist in the birthing phase, she could end up with a surgical birth.

Foetology experts are now saying that the disorientation that a baby experiences when his mother has accepted drugs can result in disconnection between mother and baby and cause a long-term feeling of abandonment on the part of the baby. Epidurals, in addition to causing dysfunction in the birthing process, can also cause a woman to run a fever. If this occurs, there is very little remedy except to get the baby born quickly.

If there is talk of induction, turn to the suggested natural means of bringing on labour in the next chapter. Don't dismiss these natural means of initiation, especially professional acupuncture, chiropractic and acupressure. If you are already in labour, but are being offered augmentation, ask for time to be able to use some of the same natural methods used to initiate labour. Ask for privacy so you can use natural methods – hugs before drugs. As long as indications point to a healthy, strong baby and you are in no danger, be willing to protect your baby from the assault of drugs.

It is important for parents to meet all diagnoses and recommendations with curiosity. They should pause and consider the effects upon the mother and the baby, as well as the overall impact of the birthing experience. It is sometimes difficult for medical care providers, accustomed to directing and playing an active role in birthing, to adjust to waiting and "standing by" in the event that they are needed. But if this is how you see your labour advancing, then this is what you should insist on.

Mothers, hold on to your bag of waters.
It is there for a reason.

WILLIAM SEARS AND MARTHA SEARS, *THE BIRTH BOOK*

When Nature Needs Assistance

While simply going beyond your due date is not by itself cause to bring about medical intervention, on rare occasions, a medically risky situation could occur in late pregnancy that should not be brushed aside or ignored as being "nothing". If you experience any of the signals listed below, call your care provider at the earliest possible time. Let your caregiver decide if, indeed, it is nothing or whether your condition requires medical attention.

Such instances include:

- Premature labour (three or more weeks early)
- Diminished foetal motion for more than six hours
- A *prolonged* period of time from release of the membrane without the natural start of labour
- Persistent and severe headaches – possibly elevated blood pressure
- A strong odor, colour or significant amount of meconium (greenish-brown, tarlike substance) in the amniotic fluid
- Excessive vaginal bleeding
- Evidence of a prolapsed cord (Get off your feet, raise your buttocks and call an ambulance.)
- Indication of infection or fever
- Persistent or excessive vomiting or diarrhoea
- Dizziness or blurred vision
- Severe swelling of hands, face, ankles or feet
- Considerably darkened urine

INITIATING LABOUR NATURALLY

Absent these factors, your relaxed attitude can work wonders in bringing about a natural start to your labour along with safe, labour-inducing techniques that you can use naturally and easily:

Hot and spicy foods. Mexican or Italian foods with "lots of hots" have had more than occasional success in starting labour. By stirring up the digestive processes in your body, you also stir your birthing muscles and your body into action. (Ask your practitioner for the special Italian recipe.) This is a good method to combine with any of the other techniques.

Lovemaking (hugs before drugs). If your membrane hasn't released, make love. Semen contains the hormone prostaglandin, which helps to soften the cervix. Here we see nature going full circle – what entered the uterus to help make the baby can help get it out. Kissing, hugging, fondling, and gentle finger or oral nipple or clitoral stimulation triggers the hormonal connection between the breast and vagina, producing the natural oxytocin that can start uterine surges. It is helpful to bring the mother to orgasm. If the stimulation of one nipple is not sufficient to start surges, try stimulation of both nipples simultaneously. However, prolonged or vigorous nipple stimulation of both nipples is not advised as it can have an adverse effect on your baby by creating hyperstimulation.

Visualisation. While your nipple or clitoris is being stimulated, use the rosebud visualisation, focusing on the rosebud's slowly unfolding and opening. Gently direct your breath down into the vaginal region while visualising.

Walk. Walk, walk, and then walk some more.

Bath. A medium-hot bath often provides the relaxation you need. You or your partner can scoop the water over your nipples and your abdomen. If your membranes have released, take a shower, directing the hot water over your abdomen.

Fear release. Have your birth companion take you through a fear-release session similar to the one practised in class so that you can search your thoughts to see if there are any lingering fears, emotions or unresolved issues that you need to release. Locked-up emotions can make you feel uptight and cause your body to produce inhibiting catecholamine. Your tension can translate into a tense cervix, preventing the flow of your natural relaxants. If you feel you need professional help, call your HypnoBirthing instructor for an individual fear-release session or ask for a referral to a hypnotherapist. It works wonders. Use this time for talking to the baby, too.

Acupressure. An acupressurist can facilitate the natural onset of labour almost immediately and, yet, afford you the time to make whatever preparations you need. Using the services of a professional will improve your chances of having the most effective points used and of obtaining faster results. If you are inclined, you can use your own skills and follow the instructions and illustrations available in many health books that cover pressure points or reflexology. Do your homework in advance so that you can apply this method when it is needed. It can also be helpful for use during labour. Do not apply pressure to these points other than at a time when you are ready to initiate labour.

Acupuncture/auricular therapy. Like acupressure, there are points that an acupuncturist or an auricular therapist can activate for the easy and effective induction of labour. These are relatively easy procedures and offer a much smoother entry into labour. Like the acupressure points, it is important that these points not be stimulated during pregnancy except for the purpose of induction when labour is slow to start or during a labour that has slowed.

Cleanse the bowel. Often the pulsating effect of emptying the bowel can stimulate the production of prostaglandin, that hormone-like substance that thins the cervix.

a. A gentle, disposable enema unit is easily obtained from a chemist or the pharmaceutical section of your supermarket or department store. This is the gentler of the two cleansing methods and quite effective.

b. Take ½ tablespoon of either castor oil or borage oil every half hour for three doses. (This is more palatable if followed by an orange juice chaser.) Because the oil creates a pulsating action in the bowel, it stimulates the onset of labour.

When you have exhausted all these means of natural initiation of labour, and it is determined that artificial induction by Syntocinon drip is an absolute necessity, you may request that only a minimal dose be administered and that it not be increased without your consent. You will also want to ask that the Syntocinon be withdrawn once your body has taken over. Many of our mothers report that the HypnoBirthing relaxation techniques that they mastered saw them through even with an induced labour, but it should be a last resort.

Childbirth – A Labour of Love: Prelude to Labour

During those months in which your baby has been developing within your womb, she's been comforted by the closeness and warmth of the wall of the membrane that softly caresses, soothes and nestles her. Your baby has felt the gentle stimulation of the swirling waters, and she's been lulled by the subtle movement of your body. She has heard and felt the love that you offered as you talked and played together.

Birth is going to bring an abrupt ending to that safe, secure period of life within the womb. At the moment of birth, your baby will emerge from her unencumbered world into a whole new series of experiences.

What your baby feels as she makes her way into the world can be a profusion of sensory encounters that can help make the baby's transition easy or cause her to tremble, jerk and cringe in fear. The experience can leave your baby with a birth memory that will affect her entire life, her personality and her spirit.

The baby startles as she takes that first breath on her own, feels air brushing across her skin, and bristles to the roughness of fabric used to rub the protective vernix from her body.

The manner in which you labour and birth, and the atmosphere into which your baby is born, should offer the same love and care that you provided as you carried him. You can assure that your baby's initial adjustment into his new surroundings is made as gentle as possible by planning and directing the course and manner of the birthing so that the welcome your baby receives is, indeed, a **labour of love**.

The environment during your birthing should be filled with the same relaxed confidence that presently surrounds your pregnancy, as well as the calm and peace that will be prevalent during the first stage of your labour. The birthing atmosphere should be free of profuse rushing, cumbersome "setting up", unnecessary medical staff, bright lights and careless, sometimes even violent, procedures that deny your baby's essence as a human being. There should be no loud, hurried voices telling you in cheerleader style to "Push, push, push", and "Keep it comin'; You can do it"!

Today's movies and television shows portray birth as comedic or traumatic; it doesn't have to be either. The birthing environment should have the same respect and calm as a place of worship. Great or humble, the decorum and protocol surrounding the birth of each and every baby should be conducted in a manner of reverence.

Together you bond.
Each one defined as three;
All three connected as one ...
Celebration of Life.

MARIE F. MONGAN, *BIRTH REHEARSAL*

Affirmations for Easier, Comfortable Birthing

Here are some suggested affirmations that should be listened to or read daily, especially during the last couple of months of pregnancy.

I put all fear aside as I prepare for the birth of my baby.
I am relaxed and happy that my baby is coming to me.
I am focused on a smooth, easy birth.
I trust my body, and I follow its lead.
My mind is relaxed; my body is relaxed.
I feel confident; I feel safe; I feel secure.
My muscles work in complete harmony to make birthing easier.
I feel a natural tranquillity flowing through my body.
I relax as we move quickly and easily through each phase of birth.
My cervix opens outward and allows my baby to ease down.
My baby is perfectly positioned for every phase of labour.
I fully relax and turn my birthing over to nature.
I see my baby coming smoothly from my womb.
My baby's birth will be easy because I am so relaxed.
I breathe correctly and eliminate tension.
As my labour advances, I go more deeply to where my baby is.
I feel my body gently sway with relaxation.
I turn my birthing over to my baby and my body.
I see my breath filling a magnificent balloon.
I am prepared to meet whatever turn my birthing takes.
The tissues in my birth path are pink and healthy.
My baby moves gently along in its journey.
My baby is positioned perfectly for a smooth, easy birth.
Each surge of my body brings my baby closer to me.
I deepen my relaxation as I move further into labour.

My body remains still and limp and relaxed.
I meet each surge only with my breath; my body is at ease.
I eat good, safe, nutritious food so that my baby will be healthy.
As labour advances, I bring myself into deeper relaxation.
I slowly breathe up with each surge.
I welcome my baby with happiness and joy.
I see my baby moving down past tissues that are pink and healthy.
As my baby is born, my blood vessels close to the appropriate degree.

Your birthing will unfold exactly as you see it now. You have defined your birthing in this way, and your birthing will happen as you have defined it.

MARIE F. MONGAN, *BIRTH REHEARSAL*

How the Body Works with You and for You

When a baby is "ripe" and ready, true labour will begin.

GRANTLY DICK-READ, M.D., *CHILDBIRTH WITHOUT FEAR*

From the very beginning of your pregnancy, your body has been working for you and with you in preparation for the time when your baby will be born, assuring that when the baby is ready, your body will be ready.

Your body has been taking prompts from your mind, and you have learned to prepare for the birth of your baby by releasing, relaxing and letting go. You turn your birthing over to your body and your baby, trusting that each knows how to do its job. This is the safest, most natural and most effective comfort measure you will use through your labour and birthing. An even deeper trust comes from knowing the ways in which your body works for you when you release and go with the flow and rhythm of labour.

Here is a reminder of some of the ways in which your mind and body assist in the birthing of your baby.

EARLY CHANGES

HORMONAL EFFECTS

As soon as your mind sends the message to the body that conception has taken place, your body begins to secrete hormones that gradually turn the hard, cartilaginous substance of the cervix into loose, spongy elasticity. By the time your baby is ready, the opening of your cervix is as soft as your earlobe.

VERTEX TURN

When you are calm, your uterus is relaxed, and your baby has room to respond to the pull of gravity, positioning himself properly in vertex position for birth. This usually occurs between weeks 32 and 37. It can, however, happen later than that. (See chapter entitled When Baby Is Breech.)

ENDORPHIN RELEASE

The relaxation techniques you have practised help to release endorphins. When endorphins are present from the very beginning of your labour, they inhibit the release of catecholamine, the stress hormone that causes muscles to tighten and constrict.

DURING LABOUR

RELAXIN RELEASE

The hormone relaxin is secreted to a greater degree during the latter part of labour. Relaxin contributes to birthing in several ways.

a. Allows the uterus and vaginal walls to stretch and become evenly smooth, without constricting bands or protruding tissues
b. Assists in softening the cervix and spreading the pubic region
c. Causes ligaments within the baby to relax, with joints (shoulder) becoming flexible for easier descent and birth
d. Weakens the amniotic membrane and allows it to release
e. Loosens the mother's skeletal ligaments, allowing the front pubic bone to shift forward to allow the baby to descend easily. Can also cause changes in gait that could lead to falls, sprains, tendonitis, etc. (Wear sensible shoes.)

RHYTHMIC SURGES

The longitudinal fibres of the uterus, in perfect precision, smoothly draw the lower, circular fibres of the uterus up and out of the way of the baby's head. Slow Breathing maximises the effect of the surge as it assists the vertical birthing muscles to move upward.

Relaxation and redirected focusing help to create a time distortion; the mind diverts attention and creates a sort of amnesia while the mother goes within to her birthing body and her baby.

MOULDING

The much-feared passing of the baby's head through the birth path is no more difficult than any other part of labour when you consider that there is a flexible, membranous material, much like a heavy canvas fabric (fontanels), surrounding the bones at the top and back of the baby's head. This soft substance allows the bones of the baby's skull to "mould" and overlap each other, reducing the circumference of the head and facilitating the smooth passage downward. Once the baby is born, the bones move into their normal positioning, creating the fontanel space, commonly known as the "soft spot". Until the fontanels fully close, which in some cases can take over a year for the frontal area, the soft spot is protected by the thick membrane.

NATURAL EXPULSIVE REFLEX

The Natural Expulsive Reflex (NER) of the mother's body rhythmically moves the baby down the birth path to the vaginal outlet, without the need for forced pushing. Baby's heart rate remains steady and is fully supplied with oxygen. Baby is born in comfort.

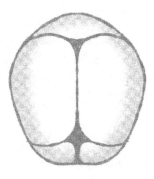

Bone Formation of Baby's Skull (Top View)

PERINEAL TONING

Pressure has a natural numbing effect. We know this when we experience the numbness that comes when we rest on a hand during sleep or when we sit on a leg for a long period of time. The perineal rim, when it is adequately softened and toned with massage, becomes numb with the pressure of the baby's head. As the baby descends, the rim of the perineum gently unfolds, allowing the baby to pass easily down and out of the vagina, just as nature intends.

PRE-LABOUR WARM-UPS

Close to the time when you are about to have your baby, it's not at all uncommon for nature to send a preview of labour in the way of uterine surges. These early surges may even trick you into thinking that actual labour has begun. What you are experiencing is, in fact, labour, but it occurs prior to that time when the cervix begins to open. By sending these early surges, nature is providing you with an opportunity to rehearse your relaxation and deepening techniques. Use them to your advantage so that they don't tire you.

Unlike actual labour, the tightening sensations are erratic and do not form a pattern. The length of the surge will differ from one time to another, and there is the absence of other signals that labour has really begun.

If you experience these tricksters, you may find that lying down, or changing your position or activity, will make the surges disappear. On the other hand, they may continue at five minutes apart for a day or even more before real labour begins. Those five-minute intervals often can be misleading.

You will want to remain in the comfort of your own home, relaxing and using some of the natural labour-inducing techniques. Resist the temptation to rush to the hospital; once you are there, you may hear the disappointing news that you have experienced little or no cervical opening. If you are in the hospital too early, you become an easy target for the suggestion of administering a vaginal gel to soften the neck of the cervix, of rupturing your membrane or starting a Syntocinon drip. Well-meaning medical caregivers, unfamiliar with your relaxation techniques, begin to get concerned about your being there for any length of time without "progressing". This is especially true if staff do not observe any of the usual signs of a labour that is "moving along".

While labour warm-ups may be annoying, especially if they linger, don't allow them to take on an importance so great as to over-shadow the joy and exhilaration of the actual birthing that is to come.

Having said that, however, I suggest that you do not brush off any different tightening sensations as mere early signals or common annoyances of pregnancy. Very often, because of their relaxed atti-tude toward birthing and an absence of fear, HypnoBirthing mums experience only a "real funny tightening in the pelvic or abdominal area" or a feeling of being constipated as the first signs of well-advanced labour. Consult with your doctor or midwife if these tightening sensations form a pattern over a longer duration and begin to occur at shorter intervals.

The Onset of Labour

Labour is usually defined as that period from the time that your cervix actually begins to thin and open until the moment that the baby is born. It is very common for the care provider to observe both thinning and opening occurring during the latter part of pregnancy. HypnoBirthers believe this is, indeed, labour even though other signs of labour have not presented themselves. This usually indicates that your body has already started the process and that the other signs will appear soon. That is good news, and it's interesting to note that this early labour-like activity is not accompanied by discomfort.

HypnoBirthing recognises only two phases of labour: the Thinning and Opening Phase, and then the actual Birthing Phase, where the baby descends as his mother assists with Birth Breathing. HypnoBirthing babies are not "pushed" into the world. They are birthed gently and naturally, the way all other animal mothers birth, with mum following the lead of her body. Immediately following birth there is the very important phase of bonding, with mum, dad and baby participating. Baby, in adjusting to his new art of breathing, recognises the scent of his parents, and handling by others should be minimal, if at all.

WHAT IS HAPPENING?

You will know that the onset of true labour has arrived when you experience uterine surges that are rhythmic – tightening and releasing in a distinct pattern. You may or may not feel your uterine surges starting. Some mums report feeling only a tightening sensation in and around the abdomen at the onset of their labour. For many HypnoBirthing mothers, these sensations are not accompanied by discomfort. As a result, they are not convinced that their labour has actually begun. Some report only that they feel constipated and need to relieve their bowels. Before or after you experience your first uterine surge, you may discover that the uterine seal that prevents bacteria from entering the uterus has dislodged. This "Birth Show" is a thick or stringy discharge that can be clear, tinged, slightly pink or bright red.

Some time at the onset of labour, or perhaps much later in your birthing, you may experience a slow leaking or a sudden gush of clear liquid from your vagina. This is an indication that the membrane surrounding your baby has released. Sometimes the release of membranes is an early sign of labour; for others, it may not occur until just before the baby is born. Babies can even be born "en caul", with the membrane surrounding them like a veil.

You may start your labour with all these signals; you may experience only one or two; you may experience none of them. The order in which they occur can differ from one woman to another and can differ with each labour for the same mother. Tune in to any unusual signs. Your baby will eventually send the message if he is, in fact, ready to be born.

If the release of your membranes is the first signal that your labour is beginning, you will want to check the fluid to be sure that it:

1) is clear with no particles, except for an occasional show of white vernix, the cheeselike covering that surrounds the baby in the sac;
2) has no colour;
3) has no putrid odour.

When the membranes release, call your care provider to report that you have examined the fluid and it meets all of the conditions mentioned above. Assure the caregiver that you wish to remain at home until your labour is under way and that you will call before leaving for the hospital. If you have hired the right caregiver, this should be the end of the conversation.

You may begin to hear of the danger of infection. While infection is a possibility, it is a very rare one, and it is not imminent. Bacteria have to be introduced into the body in order for infection to take place. As one midwife says, "The vagina is not a straw". Another advises, "The vagina is not a sponge". When you step out of the bathtub, there is no flow of water that has gathered in the vagina. One of our doctors in the US reminds his mums that bacteria are not sperm, and they don't swim.

Sometimes there is a considerable delay between the time that your membrane releases and active labour starts. This doesn't mean that something is wrong. In the event that the onset of labour is delayed, refer back to the suggestions for initiating labour naturally, starting on page 154. Women in most places in the UK are particularly fortunate in that caregivers are willing to exercise patience in waiting for labour to begin naturally. If the membranes have not released spontaneously, they are usually left to release on their own. Chances are that labour will start within 24 hours. Your temperature may be monitored, and you can politely decline vaginal examinations. It's that simple. It is not necessary that an induction procedure be initiated, barring any other indications of a need to do so. Agreeing to that first intervention or to an artificial induction in the absence of medical indication could turn your plans for a calm birth upside down.

FEELINGS YOU MAY EXPERIENCE

You'll no doubt feel a sense of excitement and joy, mixed with relief. You also may have a "ready-to-go" attitude, but you should temper that for a while. Unless you live a considerable distance from the hospital or birthing centre, remain at home for as long as you can once true labour has set in. From the time you show up at the hospital or birthing centre, your assessment will be judged by how long you have been in labour. There is also the chance that if you report and labour is not sufficiently advanced (at least 3 or more centimetres), you may have to return home. This can become a source of disappointment and frustration. If you relax, remain patient and stay at home, you may avoid these unproductive and distracting emotions.

Don't allow yourself or your birth companion to become overly caught up in the mechanics of timing and charting. You will sense when the intervals between surges are becoming shorter if you listen to your body.

Frequently, when asked, "What do you wish you had done differently?" our mothers respond, "I wish we had not gone to the hospital as early as we did".

HOW YOU MAY PARTICIPATE

The months of conditioning and practise are now paying off. Your positive attitude and confidence will allow you to remain calm and relaxed.

When your surges begin, use relaxation and Slow Breathing to increase the efficiency of each surge. If your membranes have released, it is a good idea to start relaxation, visualising the opening rosebud and breathing gently down toward your vagina. This will encourage the uterus to start surging.

If labour begins when you would normally be sleeping, capitalise on this and continue to relax and sleep. Take light foods for nutrition. Your body will need fuel to complete the task ahead, and eating will help you avoid ravenous hunger when you are in the middle of labour. The calm HypnoBirthing approach to birth inhibits secretion of catecholamines so it is likely that your digestive functioning will not be arrested. You need energy and you need to snack, drink lots of fluids to avoid dehydration and keep your bladder empty.

At your signal – usually closing your eyes – your birth companion will know that you are in surge and will stroke your arm while reciting the cues that are on the Birth Companion's Prompt Card (available from your HypnoBirthing instructor). It's not necessary to follow the prompts line by line. These are suggestions for the kinds of phrases that will assist you in remaining relaxed.

The most important factor to consider during labour may be what you sense and feel, not what you see or hear. As your birth companion gives prompts, trust your body and go deeper within each surge that you breathe up, maximising each surge to the fullest.

If you will be birthing in a hospital or a birthing centre, you will want to call your midwife and get ready to travel when your surges are approximately three and a half to four and a half minutes apart.

If you have a distance to travel, you should adjust that time to accommodate your trip.

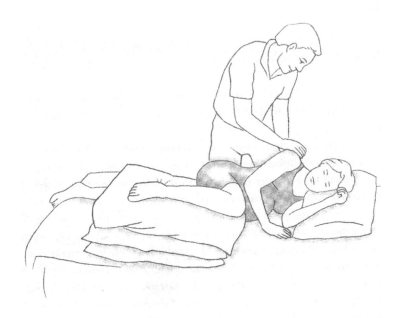

Lateral Position During Labour

Settling In at the Birth Centre or Hospital

Most hospitals prefer you to phone ahead to let the midwives know that you are ready to come in. When you arrive, if your pregnancy has been normal, you and your birth companion will be shown to a room on the labour ward. At that time you will be assigned a midwife.

In some Irish hospitals, when couples arrive they are directed to a waiting area until they are called to come in for assessment.

It is likely that the person attending you will be a labour ward midwife. In some situations this could also be a member of your team of community midwives. The midwife's visits to your room to monitor your baby's heart rate and to check your vital signs are an important part of your birthing care, not an intrusion upon it. The midwife who attends you will become an integral part of your birthing experience and, in effect, also acts as a birth companion. The warmth, care, and encouragement that the midwife extends are one of the most vivid recollections that a new mother carries with her as she leaves the hospital. These kindnesses remain a birth memory, as they should.

If you have chosen to birth your baby within a hospital setting, it is very unlikely that you will see a doctor at all. Unless there are special circumstances, the only person who will attend you is a midwife. Some hospitals have only one midwife present to attend a birthing, but often there are two midwives who may attend you. The second midwife will visit your room only when needed, so you may want to ask to meet the second midwife. This is hospital policy in most places.

If you are birthing at home, your midwife will monitor your labour in the same manner. Her assessments and your own sense of what is happening within your body will reveal to you the progress of your labour.

In addition to taking your temperature, pulse, blood pressure, and a sample of your urine, the midwife will obtain your labour history. She will palpate your abdomen to determine the position of the baby and to assess uterine activity. She will listen to the baby's heart rate to assure that all is well, and she will ask permission to perform a vaginal examination. If the examination reveals that you are still very early in your labour, it is strongly suggested that you return home until such time as your labour is more active.

Women who birth within the National Health Service are fortunate in that the guidelines set forth by NICE (National Institute for Clinical Excellence) have removed the requirement of a mandatory 20-minute monitoring on the electronic foetal monitor upon admission if the mum is low-risk and the pregnancy and labour are normal. The electronic foetal monitor (EFM) shows the foetal heart rate (FHR) and the length, intensity, and distance between your surges, and establishes a baseline for monitoring the baby's heart rate throughout labour. Unless there is indication of special circumstances, you will receive only intermittent monitoring with the EFM, and your mobility need not be limited. This is made possible with the use of a hand-held monitor called a sonicaid which is much less intrusive and can be used in whichever position you have chosen to adopt at this time.

Not all medical facilities in Ireland adhere to the NICE guidelines, however, so you may find yourself in a hospital where the 20-minute mandatory strip is still a requirement at the time of admission.

If it is determined that your labour is well established, and the initial hospital admitting procedure is complete, request that your midwife spend a couple of minutes with you to review your Birth Preference Sheets. Your birth companion can attach the door sign, a welcome acknowledgement to the staff.

At this point, you will be given time and space to settle in. You may choose to take a bath, adopt any positions that are comfortable, take a walk, drink, and do whatever feels right for you. Your birthing companion may request additional pillows and set up the CD player with your birthing music. Plan to take extra pillows from home in the event that the birthing centre is fully occupied. Be sure to use pillowcases that can be clearly identified as yours so that you don't leave them behind when you are discharged or moved.

If you are birthing in hospital there is no need for you to relinquish your clothing for the flimsy, unattractive hospital gowns that are standard hospital issue unless you want to. You may wear clothing of your own choosing. Hospital gowns, in addition to making you look like a medically needy patient, restrict your ability to wander or walk around the hospital or the grounds. Of course, at a home birth, you would be free to wear whatever you choose, to eat, walk, or shower or bathe, and enjoy the comfort of familiar surroundings. If birthing in hospital, you will want to be sure to bring snack foods with you.

PERINATAL BONDING THROUGH LABOUR

Throughout labour and birthing, you, your birth companion and your baby will be engaged in a closeness and bonding so evident that health caregivers are almost hesitant to carry out necessary monitoring for fear of intruding on the serenity of the moment. Hospital staff will be in awe as they observe you, fully calm and peaceful, responding to the touch and the voice of the birth companion as he or she sits at your side and guides you through each uterine wave. There is no doubt on the part of anyone who witnesses HypnoBirthing that the birth companion is an integral part of this wonderful experience. It is he or she who will be the person to take the lead in assuring that the atmosphere of the birthing room is dim, calm and serene. Your companion will be the advocate and spokesperson for your family, ensuring that you experience the safe, satisfying birthing that you expect.

Your companion will provide any number of supportive and comforting tasks. Most helpful are the soft, whispered prompts he gives as you and the baby move through each surge and wave of labour. The birth companion will also keep you informed about labour hallmarks. It is a form of bonding and love that may surface as it never has before.

If you have a professional labour companion/doula with you, many of the tasks that are comforting during labour will be quietly handled by her in the background. Your partner is free to devote his or her time entirely to you, and you will be aware only of how the three of you – mother, baby and birth companion – are bonding and experiencing birth together.

One of the hallmarks of a progressing labour is that your body heat begins to rise sometime during the thinning and opening phase of labour. Your birth companion will be there to gently wipe your forehead, neck and shoulders with a cool and refreshing moist cloth that has been surreptitiously provided by the labour companion, if you have one. The birth companion will see that you are comfortable, with an adequate number of pillows beneath your head, back or legs. Looking after your needs for drinks or snacks, turning the birthing music tape, seeing that there are no unnecessary bright lights in the room, reminding you to change position from time to time and to get up and go to the bathroom are things that the birth companion, in the absence of a labour companion, will do.

High on the list of the kindnesses that the companion brings to the birthing room is the gift of touch. The soft application of Light Touch Massage, simulating the flow of gentle energy from the hand and arm through Glove Relaxation, all the while expressing love and encouragement are among the welcome ways in which the partner participates. The companion is most valuable in just "being there" with you and for you, sharing in this once-in-a-lifetime event.

The mood of the birthing room will depend mostly on your mood and your wishes. Your birth companion will be sensitive to your needs and follow your lead. If you prefer to be fully conversant between surges, less attention will need to be paid to keeping birthing-room activities subdued. The birth companion should be sure that trivial conversation is avoided unless you initiate it.

If you use Sleep Breathing and stay in relaxation between surges, your companion will request that others keep voices soft, and connect or disconnect apparatus quietly and with a minimum of flurry. As the hospital staff develops a sense of your birthing style, you will find them more than helpful. You may even find that staff members are in awe and pleased for the opportunity to be a part of your birthing.

As Labour Advances: Thinning and Opening Phase

WHAT IS HAPPENING?

The cervix is thinning. The longitudinal fibres of the uterus continue to draw back the circular fibres so that the cervix increasingly thins and opens.

You will continue to experience the wave of each surge. Your abdomen will feel as though it is surging upward, tightening and then receding back down again. These surges usually last no more than thirty-five to forty-five seconds at this point. Keeping your body limp and relaxed allows this stage to pass with little or no discomfort. Intervals between surges can vary considerably.

WHAT FEELINGS YOU MAY EXPERIENCE

Your mood during the early part of this phase will usually be light and social. If you choose, you may remain sitting or semi-sitting and conversational, or you can assume a more relaxed position. You will continue to use Slow Breathing during your uterine surges, working with each one to get the most out of it. If there are others in the room, you needn't feel that you have to entertain them; this can distract you from your birthing. The earlier you go within to your birthing body, the more easily your birthing will move along.

HOW YOU MAY PARTICIPATE

Your birthing companion will continue to prompt you with cues designed to lull your responses and remind you to step aside and give your birthing over to your baby and your body. You will listen to your birthing music, feel its flow, and go with that flow, continuing to Slow Breathe with every surge.

During and between surges, you will use your own favorite images of the Opening Rose, the Rainbow, the Sensory Control Valve, the Depthometer, and Glove Relaxation. When mums in HypnoBirthing classes ask, "What should I do?" I emphatically say, "Totally relax; drink fluids and keep your bladder emptied. Other than that, do nothing!" There is nothing you can do except release and relax. Work with your body; go with the ebb and flow of the tide. Give your birthing over to your body, communicate with your baby, and just keep out of the way. Any attempt to "do something" means that you are actually resisting the way in which your body is working.

Clutching, clenching or curling up in a foetal position all create tension in your body that is counterproductive. You will also want to avoid getting caught up in activities and options that hospital staff will offer with kind intentions (unless those activities or options appeal to you). Mothers frequently say that suggestions that they take walks, spend time in a rocker or "get things moving" distracted them and broke their deep level of relaxation.

Many doctors and midwives recommend that women in labour walk. The belief is that when a woman is in an upright position, she is better able to utilise the effects of gravity to help the baby move down into the pelvis. The pressure of the baby's head against the cervix is believed to encourage dilation. It is also thought that standing expands the pelvic outlet through which the baby's head passes first. In 1997, a study in Texas, conducted through the University of Texas Southwestern Medical Center, however, found that there were no significant differences between the length of labour of women who walked and those who remained sitting, relaxing or resting. I have never observed animal mothers walking halls. Instead, they seem to go deeper into relaxation. HypnoBirthing mothers find that their cervixes seem to open more easily and quickly as a result of giving those muscles the necessary relaxation and oxygenated blood flow needed to open.

If you feel that you would like to walk, then do so, but not because you are being pressured to get on your feet and get those muscles moving.

Attempting to overcome or manipulate labour can cause fatigue and discouragement. Reverting to breathing that requires huffing and puffing or "blowing it away" simply saps the energy that you need to reserve for the time when you give those final downward breaths that will bring your baby into the world. If you have spent a sufficient amount of time conditioning your mind and body, the art will be there for you. Follow the techniques that you learned, and trust in yourself and your body's ability to birth. You'll be fresh, alert and fully energised when that wonderful moment of birth arrives.

"TUBBERS"

I spoke to a labour and birthing nurse recently who couldn't rave enough about how successful her "tubbers" were at combining HypnoBirthing and waterbirthing. We are seeing many women choose the comfort and ease of waterbirthing. It is an extraordinarily good complement to HypnoBirthing, enhancing your relaxation and allowing the baby to be born into an environment that makes for an easy transition from life within the womb to air breathing. There is no doubt about the merit of the weightlessness and buoyancy that water provides. When women use this combination, their minds are free and relaxed, and their bodies are better able to benefit from the softening effect that water has on the birthing muscles and on the folds of the perineum. One therapy contributes to the efficacy of the other.

When muscles are sore or tense, we naturally turn to a tub of water to soothe them. Advertising experts frequently use the image of a woman in an elegant, designer bathtub to sell any number of products. The association between water and sensuality is also not wasted on couples who are birthing. We often use a bath to calm a fretful or sick child. That's because it is understood that water gives us a feeling of pleasure, contentment and well-being. Water will help this phase of labour pass in a way that is beyond comparison.

Barbara Harper, founder of Waterbirth International, states that when women labour and birth in water, there is a decided increase in the production of endorphins and natural oxytocin. Many mums are better able to go deeper into their birthing bodies with the help of a soothing, relaxing tub of water. I have seen women actually luxuriate in a birthing pool. One woman smiled and sang softly through her surges while in water.

Women and birth attendants need to move past the vast amount of misinformation and bias concerning waterbirth and get the facts. Many new hospitals are including birthing tubs in their plans for their birthing units. Others are installing them into existing units.

We enthusiastically suggest it. If your birthing facility does not have a birthing tub, there are many places where tubs can be rented, and many of our HypnoBirthing families do that for home or hospital birthings. Your practitioner will help you locate a source for a birthing tub or pool.

Slow or Resting Labour

Prepare for a no-fault birth ...
If you confidently participate in all the decisions made
during your labour and delivery – even those that were not
in your birth plan – you are likely to look upon your birth
with no blame and no regrets.

WILLIAM SEARS AND MARTHA SEARS, *THE BIRTH BOOK*

The best way to manage a slowed or resting labour is to meet it with patience. Most HypnoBirthing families are better able to do that because they respectfully decline to use an Electronic Foetal Monitor (EFM) except intermittently. Most hospitals and birthing centres subscribe to the use of EFMs only when there are special circumstances.

A resting labour later does not mean that immediate steps need to be taken to restart the labour. Nature will have its way, and calm is what you need. After experiencing the calm of a nap, many mothers resume an active and even accelerated labour.

Ask for time to be able to use some of the same natural methods used to initiate or restart a resting labour. Ask for privacy so you can use natural methods – hugs before drugs. As long as indications point to a healthy, strong baby and you are in no danger, be willing to protect your baby from the assault of drugs.

Occasionally, when a mother accepts the suggestion of rupturing her membranes or of using a Syntocinon drip, her labour does not move along more rapidly. Perhaps her body is being prompted into a labour that it is not quite ready for.

It is important for parents to meet all suggestions with curiosity. In the absence of a true medical urgency, the family should pause and consider the effects upon the mother and the baby, as well as the overall impact of the birthing experience. It is sometimes difficult for medical care providers, accustomed to directing and playing an active role in birthing, to adjust to waiting and "standing by" in the event that they are needed. But if this is how you see your labour advancing, this is what you should insist on.

PASSING TIME THROUGH LABOUR

In addition to employing some of the suggestions in the section on inducing labour naturally, there are several ways in which you can pass time during a slow or resting labour that actually enhance your comfort and contribute to the opening and spreading of the pelvic area. For example:

The Birth Ball: The birth ball serves many purposes: It can offer you an alternative to remaining in bed during a prolonged labour; it is an excellent prop for you to support yourself by the side of your bed while your birthing companion applies Light Touch Massage; and it relaxes the pelvic muscles. Many hospitals provide birth balls for labouring mothers. Feel free to request one or bring your own. They're fun and so beneficial.

Tub or Jacuzzi: The benefits of the tub or Jacuzzi have already been explained. Many mothers delight in spending a good deal of time in them if their labours are taking time. If you are using a regular tub rather than a special birthing tub, you'll find that the depth of the water is rather shallow. In order to derive the most benefit from your stint in the tub, place a towel from the tips of your nipples down to your thighs to keep the protruding parts of your body warm. While gently scooping water over your body, your birthing companion can recite the usual prompts during your surges.

Shower: A warm shower, with the water directed to your abdomen, is also a good way to pass time and gives the effect of effleurage.

Humour: The breathing produced by laughter is one of the best means of relaxing. Pack several pieces of humourous reading. Many

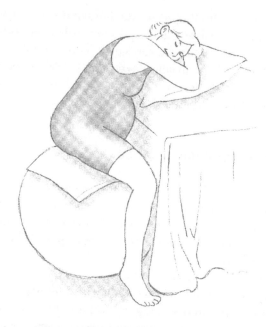

Labouring Mother Resting on a Birth Ball

of the "humour" sections of *Reader's Digest* provide an excellent source of short, amusing stories and quips. Humour increases the production of endorphins, which, in turn, block the introduction of catecholamine.

Nipple Stimulation: The stimulation of one or both nipples triggers the hormonal connection between the breast and the vagina, producing your body's natural oxytocin that can enhance your uterine surges. Ask for the privacy to be able to use nipple stimulation. Your medical caregivers will be neither surprised nor embarrassed at your request.

Light Touch Massage: Light Touch Massage, described in an earlier chapter, is among the exercises that you will want to familiarise yourself with. Your HypnoBirthing practitioner will supply you with specific instructions for the massage. Here again, we have a wonderful source of endorphin production.

Walking: This is another advantage to keeping your own clothes. Walking around the birthing unit, the hospital or even the grounds is an excellent way to pass time in labour. Fresh air has been known to work wonders. The change of scenery often relieves some of the tension that can be felt when there seems to be concern about restarting labour.

IF LABOUR WEAKENS

There may come a time when all accommodation to your wishes has been extended, but for some reason, an obvious pattern of decreased or severely weakened uterine activity forms, and your baby is not weathering it well. In such an instance, it may be determined that your birthing needs medical assistance.

In this kind of situation, you will find that your relaxed HypnoBirthing attitude and techniques can still help you through whatever turn your birthing may take. Understanding the need for medical intervention and, along with your birth companion, being a part of the decision-making team will help you accede to whatever preparations need to be made. You will remain calm and in control of your circumstances. This is HypnoBirthing.

Nearing Completion

WHAT IS HAPPENING?

You are reaching the end of the thinning and opening phase. Your surges are closer, stronger and more beneficial. The wall of your cervix has completely thinned, and the cervix is continuing to open sufficiently to allow the baby to begin to move down. When this happens, your body sends a message that it's time to change from Slow Breathing to Birth Breathing – the gentle, but firm, breathing down that will help you to bypass lengthy, difficult and fatiguing "pushing" techniques used by other methods.

Time distortion usually sets in, and you lose track of time. You will be more aware of the working of your uterus with waves rising almost as though your birthing body is separate from the rest of your body; you may or may not be aware that the surges are becoming longer and higher. As you breathe each one up to the fullest, they become more efficient. The touch and voice of your birth companion will guide you through each surge. Your journey becomes more encouraging, as labour from this point can move along very quickly, especially as you deepen your relaxation.

You drift into an almost amnesiac state, focusing on your birthing experience. You are able to entirely shut out distractions and mentally go within to your baby. At the end of this phase, as your cervix becomes fully opened, you will feel the fullness within your body and, unless you experience a resting time, you will instinctively feel the need to change your breathing pattern to the downward Birth Breathing to assist the baby in his descent.

HALLMARKS OF LABOUR

During this period, you will probably experience at least one or more of the hallmarks of labour – those milestones that tell you that your labour is moving along. They are all very natural and good messages from your body. Your birth companion will remind you of the hallmarks as you pass each one. It's exciting.

- Your body heat will rise and/or drop alternately. One minute you will be kicking off bedding; in another you'll be requesting a warmed blanket.
- When you get up to empty your bladder, there will be a spot of blood on the Chux pad that was beneath you. The body is directing its efforts downward.
- You may begin to hiccup, burp, feel nauseated or even vomit as your diaphragm has an initial reaction to the lower pulsations in your body that will soon move your baby down to birth. The good news is that it doesn't last long. (It happens rarely with HypnoBirthing mums because their bodies are calm and not in tumult.)
- Regardless of how calmly and well you have approached your birthing, you may all of a sudden feel the need "to escape". Even a mum who is having a fantastic birthing has been known to express the thought, "I don't think I want to do this any longer" or "I can't do this anymore". This last hallmark is one of the most exciting. It means that the birth of your baby is right around the corner. Your birth companion will remind you of this hallmark, and the mood changes for everyone in the room. Your baby is almost here.

WHAT FEELINGS YOU MAY EXPERIENCE

Your mood will remain calm and nearly euphoric. Your peaceful, relaxed state will turn into an almost fuzzy mood, where you will hear everything that is going on around you, but you'll not care to respond. You may go through this final phase of opening in an almost dreamlike state. Nature's amnesia will lull you so that you seem to drift in and out of alertness. It becomes even easier to place your awareness only on your baby and your birthing body.

As time distortion clicks in, the length of the surge will be distorted, and your time consciousness will fade. Twenty minutes will, indeed, seem like five. This is nature's way of helping you remain placid and serene. At the end of this phase, your shift to Birth Breathing will give you a feeling of well-being, as you and your baby work together.

HOW YOU MAY PARTICIPATE

At this time, you really settle into birthing. Your conversant stage has passed, and you are easing into the business of having a baby. Deep relaxation and a thoroughly limp body help you to block out your surroundings and go even further within to your baby.

By this time, many women have already adopted a lateral position. If you choose to stay on your back, your birthing companion needs to be sure that the head of the bed is elevated so that you are not lying flat. Lying flat can limit the supply of oxygen to your baby. Your birthing companion will help you to adjust your position if you slip down in the bed.

With deepened relaxation, you let go and let your baby and your body do what each can do best during this time. You will continue to breathe up with your uterine surges until your cervix opens, but it will seem almost effortless. With the signal of downward lower fullness, you will know instinctively that it is time to change your breathing to Birth Breathing. Your birth companion will assure staff that you are not going to push at this point and it is safe for you to change to a Birth Breath.

With no effort, you move closer to a place of utter comfort, moving in harmony with your body.

When your body sends the message that it is time to begin to nudge your baby down, you will follow the lead of your body and work with the shift of your pulsations that now direct your breathing downward in contrast to the upward breathing that you have been doing up until now. Often this is all accomplished with little notice, as the birthing mother continues to work with her surges quietly and serenely without changing position.

Your birthing companions should take turns going for food during this phase of your birthing. You should not be alone, even though you may appear to be perfectly relaxed and simply resting. That look can be deceiving, as few others are aware that you are breathing your baby down to the vaginal outlet.

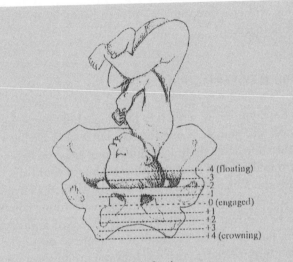

-4 (floating)
-3
-2
-1
0 (engaged)
+1
+2
+3
+4 (crowning)

Pelvic Station

The location of the baby's head within the pelvic region is measured by what is known as the Pelvic Station. You will hear reference to the Pelvic Station both before and during your birthing. As the baby journeys downward, his progress may be explained to you as being at -1 or +1 or +2. Positive numbers are below the midsection of the pelvis; negative numbers are above the midsection. The measure is determined by where the "presenting part" or top of the baby's head is. If you are told that the head is high, it means that the position is still in the minus level. The head is said to be engaged when the head is at 0.

Every child is unique. Every child must pass through the same stages, leading from an enclosed world to the open one, from being folded in on itself to reaching outward.

FREDERICK LEBOYER, M.D., *BIRTH WITHOUT VIOLENCE*

Experiencing Birth:
Breathing Love, Bringing Life

WHAT IS HAPPENING?

What is happening is **Birth!** Your baby gradually descends to the rim of the perineum, and the baby's head becomes visible (crowning). With the head nearly or fully crowned, you are ready now to give those final few breaths that will bring the baby past the perineal rim and into the world. After birth, your baby is placed immediately on the skin of your abdomen or lower chest for embrace and bonding with you and your birth companion. When the umbilical cord stops pulsating, the cord will be cut, and you, your baby and your birthing companion continue to bond.

FEELINGS YOU MAY EXPERIENCE

You will feel excitement and a bit of relief as you realise that shortly you will **birth** your baby.

Instinctively you have felt your body telling you that the change to Birth Breathing is appropriate. Instead of breathing up, as you have been doing with Slow Breathing, you now feel an urge to breath down with each surge. When the baby's descent is nearly over, you will experience a sense of extreme fullness just above the pubic area as your baby occupies the lower birth path. Your vagina will feel much like it wants to turn outward, spilling its precious content out.

HOW YOU MAY PARTICIPATE

Completion of the opening phase doesn't need to mean the onslaught of a sudden flurry of activity, confusion or additional staff on the scene. It is important that you avoid any attempt to force or rush this stage. The descent of your baby can be experienced as calmly as your first stage of labour. Many times, HypnoBirthing mums just allow this phase to begin almost unnoticed, as they remain in the position of their choice and just allow the birthing phase to play out, calmly and gently. Because there is no noticeable change in your behaviour, only the most trained eye will detect that you are birthing your baby.

It's common for hospital staff to become genuinely enthusiastic when you near completion of the opening phase, as they anticipate your actively "pushing" your baby down to crowning. The moves that fall into place at this time should follow the requests you expressed in your birth preferences. You don't want to find yourself caught up in procedures that are different from what you have anticipated. Your birth companion will express your preference for "mother-directed" breathing down through this stage and will assist you calmly with prompts that suggest a smooth, easy descent.

"Pushing your baby out" is a rude concept that has no place in gentle birthing. It is usually counterproductive and is actually a detriment, causing the vaginal sphincters to close ahead of the descending baby. It creates an atmosphere of stress for all involved. Very recent studies suggest that forced pushing over a long period of time can be harmful to a birthing mother and do damage to her pelvic floor.

Strong, forced pushing while other people prompt you will confuse, frustrate and tire you. It also causes your baby to experience emotional and physical trauma, as she is pressed against the walls of a resistant passage that is not yet receptive to her journey. Stories of exhaustive pushing that extends over hours bear out the fact that the baby will descend when she and the birth path are ready.

The wave of the lower body is designed to expel as each surge moves the baby farther down the birth path. These soft, expulsive pulsations of your body will do their job more quickly if left uninterrupted and allowed to function as nature intended. Many times, this can be achieved with little or no notice of others. Contented, relaxed and still in an amnesiac state, showing very little effort, you remain in a deepened resting mode. Often, the first time a mother lets the people attending her know what is happening is when she says, "I'm ready". This frequently means that the baby has totally descended down the birth path and is ready with just a few visible breaths to be born.

The more nature is able to take its course, the less likely you are to need an episiotomy. In the same way that the neck of the cervix needed to be gradually thinned and opened, the thick rim of the perineum needs to gradually thin and unfold through each surge by natural pressure of the baby's head until, at last, the folds open fully to allow the baby's head to pass through. It appears to be a slow unravelling, but, to the contrary, it is more swiftly accomplished with Birth Breathing than by any other means. HypnoBirthing mums talk of three or four Birth Breaths to bring the baby past the perineum and out.

Birth Breathing is the opposite of Slow Breathing, where you drew the surge up and worked with the upward wave. Now, instead of breathing up, you will take in a short, deep breath and breathe down. Your birthing companion will prompt you to direct your breath and love downward to help your baby move smoothly down to crowning. As you exhale, breathe down and visualise the opening of your vagina, like the petals of a rose, folding outward as your baby moves to the perineal rim.

If the move is going smoothly, you may choose to remain in a lateral position and simply breathe down until the baby's head is visible, or you may wish to adopt the Slanted "J" position, *being sure to rest just above your tailbone* to allow the baby plenty of room to move out.

If your baby needs some help in moving down smoothly, you may want to adopt some of the positions that are described and illustrated in the chapter entitled Positions for the Birthing Phase. Some of the recommended positions are designed to help the muscles and pelvic structure to spread and open more freely. Many of the positions call for your birth companion to assist you so that the two of you can take part in your baby's birth together.

You should be informed of the first appearances of your baby's head in a calm manner. There is a tendency for those in attendance to begin to direct this phase with loud, animated cheers. I stress that birthing is not an athletic event. Voices should not be raised. This is as much for your baby as for you. Your baby hears every sound; the sounds that he hears should not frighten him.

WHAT YOU WILL FEEL

There is no need for discomfort during the birthing phase of labour. The cervix has already thinned and opened, and now the gradual descent of the baby is conducted in such a way that there is no strain on the tissues and sphincters of the birth path. Movies and television notwithstanding, if this descent is completed as you have practised, there is no reason for pain or any other sensation. Most women experience this birthing phase calmly as they breathe down and ultimately help the baby to emerge. There is no doubt that this is the most beautiful time of birthing. This is the culmination of everything you've planned and waited for over the last nine months.

BIRTH BREATHING

For a good portion of the birthing phase, your body and baby will be working in harmony as the Natural Expulsive Reflex (NER) takes over and moves your baby down the birth path. You will assist by using the breathing technique that you have been practising for some time. Once your baby's head becomes visible, you will continue to use this downward nudge breath until the baby is gently breathed past the opening folds of the perineum and emerges in birth. This stage cannot be taken lightly if you wish to birth easily and efficiently. Just as you needed to practise Slow Breathing to bring yourself past the thinning and opening phase, you will need to practise Birth Breath. While in labour, you will follow your body's lead and work with it when you feel the onset of a surge. Here are some helpful hints:

- The best place to practise this breathing style is on the toilet as you are moving your bowels. Become aware of the pulsations that move the stool down and out. Your breaths are short intakes with gentle nudging breaths downward – nothing forceful. Practising in this way will show you that it actually accomplishes the task more easily and quickly.

- Your eyes may remain closed if you choose to stay in deep relaxation through this period. Since you will not be forcefully pushing, there is no need for you to keep your eyes open to avoid tearing the tiny blood vessels in your eyes.

- Placing the tip of your tongue at the place where your front teeth and palate meet will help your lower jaw to recede so that you remain free of tension in your mouth and jaw area. This will also help to relax the vaginal outlet.

- When you feel the onset of a surge, follow it. Take in a short, but deep, breath through your nose and direct the energy of that breath to the lower back of your throat and down through your body behind your baby in the form of a "J" – down and forward. Allow all the muscles in your vaginal area to open as though you were letting the breath out through them or moving your bowels. Don't ride out or hang on to a breath beyond its effectiveness and don't allow those lower muscles to tighten.

- Repeat this process by taking in another short, deep breath and breathe down in the same pattern as above – and then another.

- Repeat this motion several times with each surge as your body leads you through this part of birthing your baby down to crowning. Continue to work with your body as long as it is still surging. Breathing down only once during a surge can cause you to lose the effectiveness of the surge, prolong the birthing time and waste your energy.

- Firmly direct your breathing down through your body. Don't let the thrust of your breath escape through your mouth. These are not shallow breaths, but they are also not strenuous. These are deep breaths, with the energy of the breath going right down to your vagina.

- You may experience the sensation of needing to move your bowels, and that is exactly the region to which you need to direct the thrust of your breath. That is the reason we ask you to practise on the toilet.

- With the exhalation of each breath, your birthing companion will prompt you to breathe love and energy down to your baby, to open the path and to nudge your baby down to birth.

Your baby is now ready to come out and must be allowed to come easily. The head births first; the vulva gradually distends without discomfort; the baby's body emerges, often requiring only more gentle bearing down.

Positions for the Birthing Phase

Birth is not an athletic event, and there is no need to become involved with gymnastics-like positions as you birth your baby. Just as you calmly experienced the opening and thinning phase of your labour, the time you spend in birthing your baby can be equally as calm if you maintain control over what is happening and resist the early attempts of others to "take charge". Your breathing will be mother-directed Birth Breathing that will assist you in gently bringing about the descent of your baby.

Nothing needs to change until the baby's descent is complete, and he is crowning. The important factor in birthing is how comfortable you feel in the birthing position that you choose and how you feel you can best assist in the baby's emergence.

There are several positions that you can adopt during the birthing phase of labour that actually enhance the widening of the birth path and shorten this phase of labour. They also reduce the likelihood of an episiotomy.

For many years the most common positions used for birthing were those preferred by the medical caregivers – chosen for the ease of technical applications and instruments. While the methodology changed, the positions remained the same with women on their backs in a lithotomic position, their legs being folded back or elevated in any number of ways. Today with HypnoBirthings, we are seeing large numbers of caregivers who are responsive to the birthing mother's lead, and they attend from whatever position the mother is comfortable in or feels she wants to assume. The supine position, nearly flat on your back and with feet in stirrups, is most assuredly a thing of the past, and rightly so. It is the least effective and increases the likelihood of having an episiotomy.

The positions described and illustrated here may require practise with your birth companion to tone your legs or your arms, but you will value this well-spent practise when you are birthing.

Semi-Reclining (Slanted "J"): When your baby is coming smoothly and easily, this very frequently used position will help you to maintain your deep relaxation during the time that you are breathing your baby down. The slanted "J" places you on a bed, *resting just above our tailbone*, with pillows behind your head, shoulders and back. The head of the bed is elevated to a 45-degree angle. Usually your legs are gently spread apart with a pillow under each knee. This position can be modified into a semi-squatting position by placing your ankles against your buttocks and spreading your legs and feet wide and to the side. This position also widens and stretches the pelvic area.

Lateral: You may be quite accustomed to this position, as many mothers tell us that they have been sleeping in a variation of the Lateral position for some time. This is also the position that many mums prefer during relaxation sessions. Birthing in the Lateral position is a frequent choice because of the ease with which you are able to move smoothly from the opening phase directly into breathing your baby down through the birth path without having to change positions. For birthing, the leg that you rested on pillows during labour is held up slightly to provide clear access to the vaginal outlet once the baby has completely descended. Until that time, you may remain just as you are with legs on pillows.

Leaping Frog: This position is an easy form of squatting, which some experts believe is one of the most effective positions for bringing your baby into the world. While squatting on your toes, place your arms inside or outside of your legs and support yourself on your hands. When your arms are outside and slightly back at the side of your hips, it is easy to spread your legs wide and allows you a clear view of your baby's birth. Another advantage of the Leaping Frog with arms outside is that your entire lower pelvic area is suspended, leaving your baby to finally emerge without pressure from other parts of your body. This position widens the vaginal opening, utilises the effect of gravity, shortens the birth path, and places the lower body up and away from any pressure. If you think you may

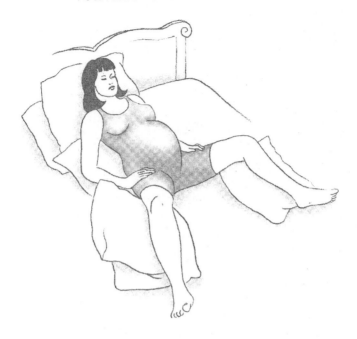

Semi-Reclining Position

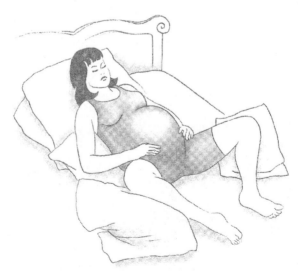

Semi-Reclining Position Modified

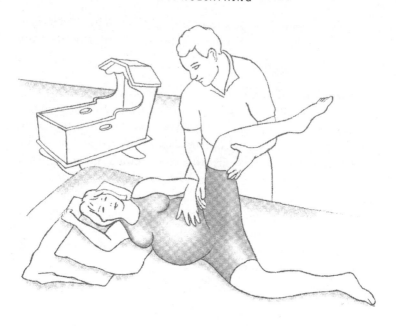

Lateral Position

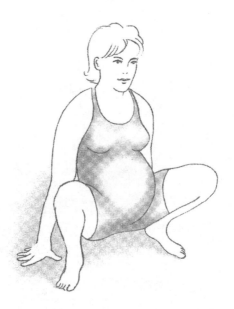

The Leaping Frog

utilise the Leaping Frog position, you will want to practise it regularly to strengthen your arm muscles, but it is worth any effort you may put into it.

Supported Squat: With all of the advantages of the Leaping Frog position, your baby can easily emerge in birth with you assuming the Supported Squat position. Instead of using your arms to support your body, you can nicely support yourself by resting your arms, bent at the elbows, on your birth companion's upper leg while he/she sits at the edge of a low chair if you are birthing at home, or at the edge of the lowered hospital bed if you are at a birthing facility. This position allows you to lean back against your partner between surges and readily return to the position when a new surge comes. From this position your baby can birth with the same advantages of using the Leaping Frog position.

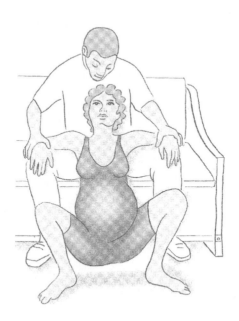

The Supported Squat Position

Toilet Sitting: Many women find a great deal of comfort in Toilet Sitting while they are still in the opening phase and while breathing their baby down. The body naturally responds to this position as it is conditioned to release and let go when toileting. This is a familiar position and location for HypnoBirthing mums because they are advised to practise their Birth Breathing while they are sitting on the toilet, moving their bowels. The two sets of muscles are closely related, and the Natural Expulsive Reflex (NER) present in birthing is supported by Birth Breathing. This position can offer the kind of spread that helps your pelvic area, opens your vagina, utilises gravity and relieves you from having to support yourself on your legs. Just place a pillow or two behind your back and relax. As you near the crowning period, you will have to assume another of the birthing positions in order to safely birth your baby.

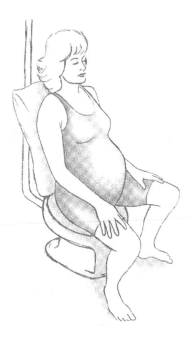

Toilet Sitting

Birthing Stool: The Birthing Stool has many of the same advantages as Toilet Sitting in that it widens the pelvic area and shortens the birth path. Additionally, it allows the mum to have the security and confidence that comes from being able to lean back against her partner between surges. Like Toilet Sitting, this is a familiar position for the birthing mother because she used this to practise Birth Breathing.

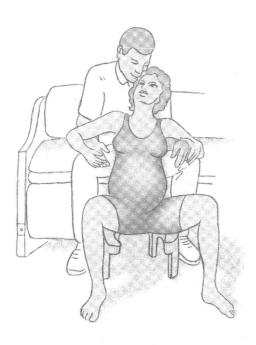

Birthing Stool

Hands-and-Knees: This position can easily be assumed from the Leaping Frog position by simply moving forward on your hands and bringing the lower part of your body up and forward over your knees in an all-fours stance. In this position, you will be on all fours leaning your weight on your knees and on your palms. This position is frequently used by women who have hired midwives as their birth attendants. This is a good position to assume if your baby needs an assist to get into an optimal position for emerging. You can

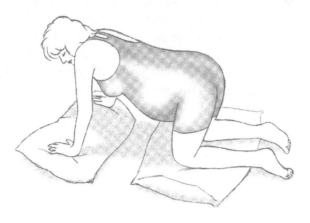

Hands-and-Knees Position

also enjoy a modified version of the Hands-and-Knees position by leaning over a birthing ball. Hospital beds can sometimes be adjusted to accommodate this position. If you are birthing at home, kneeling on a pillow with your arms and upper body supported on another pillow on a chair will give the same effect.

Supported Stand: The Supported Stand utilises the advantages of gravity in helping the baby move down the birth path. It involves having your partner support himself by leaning against a wall and extending his arms. You can support yourself on his arms by leaning back against him while you rest your underarms on his lower arms. You both will want to flex your legs at the knees slightly.

Polar Bear: While the Polar Bear position is not a birthing position, it can be helpful if the baby is found to be in a less than optimal position for emergence. This favourable position can be assumed from a Hands-and-Knees position by placing your forearms on the floor in front of you and resting your forehead on your hands. Both the Polar Bear and the Hands-and-Knees position allow your baby to move back from the lower pelvic area and turn to a more beneficial position for birthing if this is needed.

If the baby does need an assist to move to a more optimal position, the Rebozo technique can be nicely utilised while mum is in

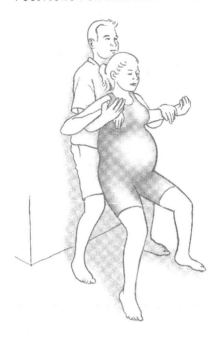

Supported Stand Position

the Polar Bear position. The technique, developed by midwife Guadalupe Trueba, is well known in Mexico and is fast making its way into birthing rooms in the United States. It is simply done by placing a long scarf under the mother's abdomen at the area of the pelvic region and lifting upward. This manoeuvre lifts the baby out of the present position and provides him with an opportunity to, in effect, back up and return to the birth path in a more favourable position for easy birthing.

For a home birth, if a scarf is not available, a curtain, a small sheet or a tablecloth can be used with the same results. Larger sheets can become cumbersome because of their bulk. Creative nurses may be able to offer suggestions in a hospital setting.

If the baby and the mother are both strong, before agreeing to a surgical birth because the baby is not positioned optimally for birth, parents need to ask for time and the opportunity to use techniques like the Polar Bear position, the Rebozo technique and self-hypnosis with the mother coaxing the baby into a more

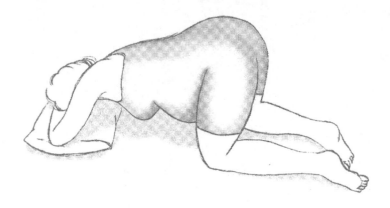

Polar Bear Position

favourable position. A malpositioned baby is not an immediate emergency unless there is indication that the mother or the baby is in distress.

Crowning and Birthing

This is the first time that you "see" the results of your labour as the tip of the baby's head becomes visible. You will feel encouraged when you reach this point. The natural pulsations of your body will slowly urge your baby forward as you continue to direct the breathing that assists your baby to crowning.

When the top of the head is fully visible, one or two more surges are usually all that is needed to gently birth the baby's head. It is amazing how easily a head can pass through the elastic perineum if you remain relaxed. Tears in the skin can be avoided if the mother has practised perineal massage and there are no rushed, violent pushes.

The birth companion will continue to help you return to a relaxed state between surges. Birthing prompts are repeated here also. The entire pelvic area should be kept as relaxed as possible. Directing your breath toward the vagina and helping the baby to move forward will help the perineum to unfold.

If everything is fine, the baby should be birthed fully before suctioning or other routines are performed, and one of the parents should receive the baby if that is their wish. The handling of the baby by someone other than a parent should be minimal and utilised only if necessary. Many caregivers today are willing to help make the baby's transition into her new surroundings less traumatic by refraining from suctioning unless there is clear indication of need. Mum, too, is spared an episiotomy unless it is absolutely necessary.

If all is normal, this is the end of the birthing phase of your labour.

BONDING

If you don't already know if your baby is a boy or a girl, you'll not have to wait long, for as soon as the baby is born, your birthing companion will announce the sex of the baby to you. You'll share this happy time together while caregivers visibly observe the baby's condition and assess mum's needs.

The baby is placed immediately on your bare chest or abdomen for bonding. Remarkably, studies called Kangaroo Mother Care, out of Australia, have found that the mother's body heat adjusts to the needs of her newborn.

The birthing companion places his hand on the baby's back to offer the security of skin-to-skin bonding that is so important during these first few moments. Handling by others should be minimal, if not absent entirely. The baby needs to feel safe among the people whose scents and energies she is most familiar with.

There is no need to rush to "clean" the baby, nor to cut the cord. It is more important for the newborn to experience skin contact with both of its parents, if possible. The vernix caseosa, that cheesy covering that makes your baby look like a channel swimmer, will simply be absorbed into the baby's skin – it is a gift from nature. Any excesses will be removed later when baby has her first bath.

You will experience an exhilaration beyond compare in these first few incredible moments as you and your birth companion touch and hold the baby, watching her begin to stretch and move and unfold, gaining a tactile sense of her new environment, one arm and one leg at a time.

Bonding during those first few precious moments of your baby's life will provide a natural high that defies description, and the feeling that you and your companion experience will remain with you for the rest of your lives. This is when the relationship that began before your baby was born is reaffirmed with actual skin-to-skin bonding – mother and father (or other birthing companion) embracing in loving union.

It is during this time that a loving relationship is affirmed, and this wonderful happening should not be rushed. Through your caresses, gaze and soft conversation, you validate your infant's acceptance and approval. The baby feels this love, and his feelings of security and self-worth are validated.

HypnoBirthing practitioners who have witnessed that first gaze when the infant's eyes meet with his parents' cite this as one of the most spiritual times in their lives as birthing educators.

Like all mammals, babies are genetically and instinctively programmed to take to the breast. You may wish to bond with your baby in this way, while the birth companion continues to support the baby's body with his hand or becomes involved with the cutting of the cord. Putting your child to the breast immediately has physical, as well as psychological, benefits. This contact and stimulation at the breast causes your uterus to begin to contract, helps to expel the placenta and appropriately closes blood vessels to avoid any possible excessive bleeding. Your midwife will offer suggestions and assistance to help you and your baby as you experience your first feeding.

Savour this time of bonding for as long as you wish and don't yield to the needs of hospital staff to carry out administrative details like weighing, measuring and cleaning. This is your new baby for whom you have been waiting for months. Take time to get acquainted. These moments can never be recaptured. It's important for you, your baby and your family.

To be sure that you are able to enjoy the wonder of these moments, the birth companion will want to talk with your attending midwife sometime during your labour to remind her of your birth preferences. Mention your wishes to have your birthing companion announce the sex of your baby and to have skin-to-skin contact with your baby, rather than have your baby wrapped in a receiving blanket. She or he will be more than happy to assist in seeing that this part of your birthing goes exactly as you wish.

Post-Birth Activities

WHAT IS HAPPENING?

Still at work for you, your body reacts to the euphoria you are feeling by stimulating the uterus into the final stage. The umbilical cord is cut after it stops pulsating. With one or two more surges, the placenta is born. You and your birth companion bond with your new baby.

From this point on, all who share this wonderful miracle experience a very enjoyable high. Often doctors and midwives who witness HypnoBirthing express awe at participating in the experience. An indefinable feeling of joy and pleasure sweeps in and takes over. You and your birthing companion may be oblivious to the activities of medical caregivers at this point as you experience getting acquainted with your new baby.

It is important that the clamping and cutting of the cord be delayed until after it stops pulsating. When the cord is prematurely cut, it abruptly cuts off the flow of blood to the baby, depriving him of that source of oxygen and of the many nutrients that will affect his health for a lifetime. Allowing the baby to take his first breaths with the continued benefit of oxygen from the placenta eases the task of taking air into his lungs once he is outside the womb. It is an easier and more comfortable introduction to breathing.

Your baby is put to the breast. HypnoBirthing babies, alert and comfortable, usually take to the breast within minutes of their birth.

Dr. Lennart Righard's *Delivery Self-Attachment* video, resulting from a study in Denmark published in 1990, shows the ability of newborns who were not medicated during labour to crawl to the mother's breast, just as other mammals do, and suckle. On the other hand, even with help, the babies whose mothers were medicated lacked the ability to crawl to the breast and were unable to suckle even with assistance.

When the cord has stopped pulsating, it is clamped. Your companion, if he or she chooses, may take part in cutting the cord, separating the baby from the cord and placenta.

The expulsion of the placenta should be allowed to occur naturally with just one or two pushes as your uterus continues to surge. You may or may not be aware of these continued surges as your placenta is birthed. These final surges help your placenta to loosen from the wall of the uterus and assist the uterus to begin to assume its normal size. Allowing your placenta to break away in this normal manner can take anywhere from five to thirty minutes. In the event that the placenta is not birthed within a reasonable amount of time, your medical caregiver may suggest a medical assist with the use of Syntometrine. However, this can be omitted if the mum requests, and a purely physiological approach may be taken. The cord should not be pulled in order to effect an extraction.

Your midwife or doctor will examine your placenta and then the abdomen to determine the "tone" of your uterus. Nursing will help the uterus return to its normal substance and size. Though episiotomies are not routine today, this would be the time for an episiotomy repair.

HOW YOU MAY PARTICIPATE

During this phase, there is really very little participation required from you. Most of the activity will centre around the medical staff's being sure that all medical procedures are complete. Your birth companion will be sure to observe that the cord is not pulled. You and your birthing companion will spend your time bonding, together, with your new baby.

Following this initial bonding, which can last up to two hours, the baby may be bathed and freshened. In some hospitals the baby is bathed right in the labour and birthing room, and the father is assisted in this special task. You will welcome this time to freshen yourself and to have your clothes and bedding changed. Very shortly the baby may be returned to you for more "get-acquainted time".

An indescribable feeling of joy, excitement and even giddiness sweeps in and takes over. Congratulations! **Your miracle is complete!**

The Fourth Trimestar

You have spent months preparing for your birth and learning skills to eliminate anxiety and discomfort, and finally the time that you have long awaited has arrived. During the time immediately following your birth and for the next three months, you will experience a dramatic transition in your current lifestyle. You are a family.

This is when you wonder why your baby did not come with operating instructions! Communication with this tiny creature who doesn't speak your language is, at best, a challenge and can, at times, seem totally frustrating. There is very little schooling that can prepare you for parenthood. It is more like "on-the-job training", twenty-four hours a day, seven days a week! That is why some people call this time period "Parent Boot Camp". It is exhilarating, confusing and wonderful all at the same time. Eventually, you, too, will become a seasoned, expert parent, able to conquer feeding, burping, nappy changing, bathing and crying, yet still have time to feed yourself, go to the bathroom and take a shower.

Some childbirth educators more affectionately call this special time a "babymoon." Much like a honeymoon, this is a time to get to know each other. This period is more frequently being referred to as the "Fourth Trimester", chiefly because there is a growing awareness that development is still going on, as the family settles in and gets used to being a family of three, rather than a couple. Take a moment now and consider this transition period from your infant's point of view. Your baby is a stranger to your world. Until his birth, he lived in a water-filled sac, never truly experiencing light, heat or hunger changes. He was calm and restful when you moved around a lot and active when you were still.

Some babies seem content in their new world, while others seem to experience the transition with a little more difficulty. Think of a time in your own experience when you left your home and travelled to a new and strange place. Did you sleep well in a strange bed those first few nights? Transitions take time. Allow your baby some time to adjust to his new life by making it as similar to his life in the womb as possible – just the three of you. The bond between you and your child will grow stronger each day.

Your entire focus should be on your baby's adjustment to his new world, and not on hosting well-wishers. How many people came with you on your honeymoon? The privacy and the moments of exploring and getting acquainted are just as important now. You all need calm and peace and bonding as much as you did before your baby's arrival.

To begin with, minimise contact with the outside world. Simplify your daily life to meet your basic needs. Wear your pyjamas all day and order in food. This is not the time to have a constant stream of co-workers, friends and relatives drop in. Guests, especially female, tend to want to hold new babies, but it needs to be remembered that babies are making a tremendous adjustment. They need to get accustomed to the scent and the touch of their parents and to become acclimatised to their new surroundings.

Allow friends and relatives to come over only if they are bringing you a meal, want to do laundry, go shopping for you or clean your house! Having these needs met makes the next leg of your journey into parenthood enjoyable and rewarding, and helps to create a transition into your new roles as parents and your infant's new role of going from pre-born to newborn.

To accommodate the well-wishers who may call, leave the details of your baby's birth date, time, weight, and so on, on your telephone's answering machine. Be sure to state that you will be happy to have visitors in a couple of weeks when you all have had a chance to become acquainted and adjusted to your new family. Turn off the ringer and the volume on the phone. It is also helpful to place a note at your door when you are resting with very much the same message.

Human babies are among the most helpless of newborns. Their instincts for survival include a strong rooting and sucking reflex. Instinct also tells them they are 100 per cent dependent on their parents. They are capable of distinguishing their parents' voices, scents and touch from those of strangers. Every day they learn about our world by how we treat them and respond to their needs. When you put down your baby, he doesn't know where you are or when you will return. Being alone, flat on his back, on a cool, firm surface with no noise surrounding him is about as unfamiliar an environment for your baby as you can get. That is why he will sleep more soundly on your chest, next to you, or in close proximity to where you are than he will if he is separated from you. From baby's perspective, separation is not an option if he wants to survive. This is how seriously your baby considers his connection to you. Remember, he probably was very happy back in the womb where all his needs were immediately met.

In spite of what some people say, you cannot spoil your baby. That is just not possible. The more you become responsive to your baby's body language and adept at interpreting his noises, the more content your baby will be, and the less he will feel the need to cry to gain your attention.

Babies cry because they need to convey a message to you. When they are not being comforted, they become confused and frightened about their chances of survival in this world. The more responsive you are to your baby's needs for touch, warmth and food, the more she will grow to be an emotionally and physically stable child, ready to achieve all those milestones of development. Meeting those needs in the early days and weeks creates the solid groundwork for trust and independence later in life.

Understanding your baby will help you minimise your own frustration and increase your enjoyment of parenting. Babies whose needs are responded to learn that they don't need to cry. There are many ways you can help your baby learn that she doesn't need to cry to get your attention. The first of these is to be responsive to the noises she makes when she first awakens. Listen for those little grunts and moans, and the smacking of her lips, as she tells you that very soon she will be fully awake and will need to be fed. Pick up your baby before she feels the need to cry, and she will learn the security of not needing to cry to get your attention.

During this "babymoon", in spite of the exhilaration that new HypnoBirthing mums feel, they can sometimes be up and sometimes be down. This is normal, and knowing this can make this time seem less erratic. Physiologically, the hormones that supported the pregnancy are rapidly decreasing, while the hormones that support lactation begin to function. These changes can make mother emotionally sensitive for a while. The cure is lots of support and rest during those early days at home. Learn to nap. Using your relaxation tapes or music from your HypnoBirthing class will help you and your baby to rest. A special HypnoParenting tape that addresses some of the feelings you are experiencing as new parents is now available through your practitioner or the HypnoBirthing Institute. It will help you realise that what you're feeling is not unusual, and it will ease your concerns.

Who is going to do all those daily chores to keep your house running smoothly? Dad? Grandma? A doula? Mums are busy enough learning to feed their infants and caring for themselves physically. Setting up your support system ahead of time for at least two weeks after the baby is born is very important. It can speed your return to feeling confident in yourself again and help avoid fatigue.

RECOMMENDATIONS FOR POSTNATAL BONDING

- As often as you can, hold the baby on the left near your heart. Babies need love and touching as much as they need nourishment. They feel at home hearing the beat of your heart.
- React to baby's communication (crying). Babies cry because something is upsetting or confusing to them as they attempt to adjust to their new existence outside of the womb.
- Make new affirmations and recite them during feeding or bathing time. Talk to your baby and caress him as much as possible; you will love every minute of it.
- Repeat as many of the prenatal bonding experiences as possible so that the same familiar sounds and interactions can help the baby adjust to his new life. Play your music tape to soothe fretful times and read some of the readings that you read while the baby was in your womb.
- Refrain from any negative expression or tone toward the baby's bodily functions – stools, spitting up, burping.
- Avoid fatigue as much as possible and don't internalise the baby's "fretfulness". Don't do battle with this little being. He is not out to see that you never get a hot meal or a good night's rest. Remember, it isn't easy for baby, either. Stay calm.

- Avoid getting stressed. This is a good time to call back the techniques of relaxation that you've become an expert at. Listen to relaxation music as often as you can, even if you pause for only a few minutes at a time. Stop for a few moments and do some Sleep Breathing to help you return to a calm state.

As hard as it may seem at times, you will actually find that these first few months will go by all too soon. You'll find yourself looking back on your baby's infancy and missing those wonderful moments when you and your baby were first getting acquainted. Very quickly the baby will pass through one stage after another and, before you know it, your baby will be a toddler. The attitude that you adopt during the early weeks will serve you well through these later challenges.

Below is a piece about that wonderful stage of growth and exploration when your child is discovering the world and its many wonders. It may help you to remember that children act like children, and it is unrealistic to think or expect that they should act like adults. They need care, guidance and love so that they can make this journey successfully. They need to be guided and loved.

'Please, Mum and Dad ...

My hands are small. I don't mean to spill my milk.

My legs are short – please slow down so I can keep up.

'Don't slap my hands when I touch something bright and pretty. I don't understand.

Please look at me when I talk to you. It lets me know you are really listening.

My feelings are tender – don't nag me all day. Let me make mistakes without feeling stupid.

Don't expect the bed I make or the picture I draw to be perfect. Just love me for trying.

Remember, I am a child, not a small adult. Sometimes I don't understand what you're saying.

I love you so much. Please love me just for being myself, not just for the things I can do.

AUTHOR UNKNOWN

Breastfeeding Is Best Feeding

Contributed by Robin Frees,
Lactation Consultant, HypnoBirthing practitioner

It is your baby's "birth" day. If you could ask your baby about the best gift he could get from you, what would that be? Your baby would want to breastfeed. So before making a decision about infant feeding, consider the following thoughts and information. Give breastfeeding a try and make an informed decision about your long-term goals for nurturing your child.

Breastfeeding is the perfect gift of love, security and health all in one simple act. Just as your womb nourished your child for nine months, now your breasts are ready to continue that connection of food and nurturing for your baby. Just as your amniotic fluid acquired tastes and smells from your diet and your infant swallowed this while in the womb, breast milk also has flavours from your diet, and after birth, your baby continues to experience many new tastes. This is a gift that money can't buy. Whether you decide to breastfeed for a few weeks, months or years, this is your first opportunity to give your baby a gift with benefits that will last a lifetime. Earlier we discussed your baby's need for connection; what better way to meet his many needs than to be held and breastfed?

In recent years, research has confirmed that breast milk is truly a unique food that cannot be duplicated. Formula is not equal to breast milk. The evidence of this fact became so overwhelming that in 1997 the American Academy of Pediatrics adopted a policy statement recommending that children receive breast milk for twelve months or more. The World Health Organisation recommendations on the priority of infant nutrition are in the following order:

1)   mother's own milk directly from the breast
2)   expressed mother's milk fed to infant another way
3)   other human milk (from a milk bank)
4)   infant formula.

One of the outstanding benefits of human milk is that it is custom-made for each infant. Mothers with premature infants make milk that is specifically composed for their infant with extra antibodies and proteins. Breast milk contains not only carbohydrates, fats and proteins, but also has growth hormones and special substances that enhance visual and brain development, as well as antibodies to fight infection. Scientists are unable to put these valuable substances into formula. Studies have shown children who breastfeed have fewer instances of ear infections, diarrhoea and upper respiratory infections. The advantages carry over into later periods in life. Adults who were breastfed have lower cholesterol and fewer occasions of heart disease. Studies have also shown that women who breastfeed have lower rates of breast cancer and cervical cancer. In addition to experiencing fewer common illnesses and diseases, breastfed children have higher IQ's.

You may not have considered the financial value of this resource that your body makes at no cost to you. If you were to bottle-feed formula to your infant for a year, it may cost between £600 and £1,500. No wonder mothers call breast milk "liquid gold". Your body provides your baby this perfect diet absolutely free.

Normally, breastfeeding is a skill that is easy for you and your baby to learn. Mothers and babies have been doing this for thousands of years. As with any skill, like dancing or driving a car, the more you do it, the better you get at it. Getting through the first couple of weeks may seem natural or, at first, seem awkward, but given time, you and your baby will enjoy this special experience more and more.

During the first couple of days your body has a small amount of early milk called colostrum. This is the time when your infant can practise latching on and sucking before the milk begins to increase in volume from teaspoons to ounces. Colostrum is an effective laxative that can help clear the meconium (baby's first stools) from your baby's system. It is also full of antibodies to protect your baby from illness. If your baby is sleepy and uninterested in eating, you can always express your colostrum onto a spoon and feed it to your baby to entice him to want to feed. Holding your baby skin-to-skin is another way for your baby to become interested in feeding. Studies show that the breast secretes a smell similar to amniotic fluid to attract the baby.

Learning a new skill is easier when someone is helping you. You didn't learn to drive a car by yourself. Remember to ask for help. Watching other mothers breastfeed before your baby is born will help you learn faster, too.

You may experience some breastfeeding challenges during the first week, but as you did during your pregnancy, keep a positive attitude toward breastfeeding. It soon becomes a gift to both mother and baby alike. If you experience discomfort, know that it is not a normal part of breastfeeding and indicates that you need attention. The earlier a problem is identified, the easier it is to solve. Lactation consultants and breastfeeding support volunteers are available in most communities. A supportive health-care provider or hospital staff will have information and can refer you to a breastfeeding expert in your area. Setting up your support system before your baby is born and learning about breastfeeding from knowledgeable sources like the Breastfeeding Network (www.breastfeedingnetwork.org.uk) can minimise problems.

If problems do occur, there are two things that you can do while you are looking for help. First, maintain your milk supply. As long as you remove milk from the breast (5–8 times/day), you will make more milk. If your baby cannot feed from the breast, remove milk with hand expression or use a breast pump. The second thing you need to do is feed your baby. You can use the milk you have expressed, or you may be advised to supplement with formula until your supply increases. A baby who is gaining weight will be eager to learn to breastfeed. Support and timely "hands-on" help will create a positive learning environment for him.

It is important for people close to the mother to be emotionally supportive of her decision to breastfeed. Many fathers and grand-parents today want to play an active role in caring for the new baby and wonder how they can be more involved if the baby is mother-fed. There are many ways they can participate in other daily activities besides feeding. Walking, holding, rocking and burping the baby after feeds can support the mother in these activities and allow the baby to get to know others in the family. While changing nappies may not be as appealing, it is another way for others to show they care! Baby's bath at the end of the day is a wonderful way for fathers to connect with their children.

Remember your reasons for learning about HypnoBirthing? You were looking for a birth experience that is calmer and safer for you and your baby – one that will give you more confidence than other experiences that your friends and relatives may have had in their birthings. The same is true with breastfeeding. Well-meaning acquaintances may have had difficulty breastfeeding because they could not find help or information when they needed it, but don't let that stop you from making this important decision for your baby. After the birth of your baby, Mother Nature assumes you will breastfeed and provides you with an abundance of milk. This is the time to go with breastfeeding and see how much you and your baby enjoy this special bond. It is a most special gift that you and your baby will surely appreciate, and it will build a bond that will last for a lifetime.

APPENDIX: BIRTH PREFERENCE SHEETS

The following pages are copies of the worksheets that your HypnoBirthing practitioner will provide for your use in designing your birth preferences. It is a good idea to complete the Birth Preference Sheets prior to touring the facility you will use for your birthing. You may wish to discuss some of the items with the person conducting your tour.

This plan has been developed for use throughout the United States and in several foreign countries. For that reason, you will find items on the plan that may not apply to you or the facility at which you will birth. Several of the items that are listed have been adopted by most hospitals and staff long ago. However, many of the requests that are routinely honoured in some geographic areas are as yet unheard-of in other areas of this country and outside of the United States. You may skip these items, mark them N/A, or extract only those that apply to your own preferences.

BIRTH PREFERENCE SHEETS

PRE-ADMISSION REQUESTS

We request:

❑ To consider artificial initiation of labour only if labour is unusually delayed and there is medical urgency.

❑ To delay artificial induction of labour for a reasonable period after the release of membranes if mother and baby show no signs of infection.

❏ To remain at home as long as possible before going to the hospital.

❏ OTHER REQUESTS: ————————————
————————————————————

FOR HOSPITAL ADMISSION

We request:

❏ The patience and understanding of caregivers to support our wish to refrain from having any practice or procedures that, in the absence of medical urgency, could unnecessarily stand in the way of our having the most natural birth possible.

❏ The opportunity to discuss our birth preferences with our assigned midwife.

❏ To return home until labour progresses if less than 4 centimetres opened and if there are no situations that warrant admission.

❏ Natural means of inducement, moving to minimum doses of artificial induction only if medically urgent.

❏ That artificial induction drugs be removed once uterus is naturally thinning and opening.

❏ To have a private labour and birthing room, subdued lighting, music and quiet tones.

To have the following persons present during my birthing:

❏ husband   ❏ other birthing companion
❏ relative   ❏ labour support person

❑ To have pictures and/or video of this important time in our lives.

❑ To have telephone calls relayed to our room.

❑ To have no telephone calls relayed – only messages.

❑ To respectfully decline to participate in the taking of pain scale information.

❑ OTHER REQUESTS: ————————————————

————————————————————————————————

DURING FIRST-STAGE LABOUR

We request:

❑ The patience and understanding of care providers to support our wish to refrain from any procedures or practices that in the absence of medical urgency could unnecessarily stand in the way of our having the most natural birth possible.

❑ To have only necessary hospital staff or cheerful observers, please.

❑ That staff refrain from references to "pain, hurt, etc." and any offer of medication or labour-enhancing procedures unless requested.

❑ Manual intermittent monitoring after pattern is established.

❑ Internal monitoring only in the event of medical urgency.

❑ Nutritional snacking if labour is prolonged.

❑ Freedom to walk and move or not walk or move during labour.

❑ To change positions and assume labour positions of choice.

❏ Minimal number of vaginal examinations – with permission – to avoid premature rupture of membranes.

❏ That labour be allowed to take its natural course without references to "moving things along" or "augmenting labour".

❏ To use natural oxytocin stimulation – nipple or clitoral stimulation – in the event of a slow or resting labour, and to be accorded the privacy to do so.

❏ To be fully apprised and consulted before the introduction of *any* medical procedure – augmentation, amniotomy, membrane stripping .

❏ To enjoy labour tub or shower.

❏ OTHER REQUESTS: ───────────────
───────────────

DURING BIRTHING

We request:

❏ The patience and understanding of care providers to support our wish to refrain from any procedures or practice that, in the absence of medical urgency, could unnecessarily stand in the way of our having the most natural birth possible.

❏ To remain in the tub for waterbirthing if available (arranged beforehand).

❏ That natural expulsive pulsations of the body be allowed to facilitate the gentle descent of the baby, with mother-directed Birth Breathing to crowning. Birth companion will offer prompts. No coaching.

❏ Use of HypnoBirthing breathing techniques – not other methods.

❏   To assume a birthing position of choice that will least likely require an episiotomy.

❏   Use of warm-oil compresses to avoid episiotomy. No perinatal massage to perineum.

❏   Episiotomy only if necessary and only after discussion.

❏   Use of topical anaesthetic for episiotomy.

❏   Videotaping of birth.

❏   To have our other children present [ ]during [ ]shortly after birth.

❏   OTHER REQUESTS: ————————————————————
————————————————————————————————————

FOLLOWING BIRTHING

We request:

❏   That father/birth companion announce sex of baby to mother if sex is unknown.

❏   That birth companion or mum receive baby if at all possible.

❏   Immediate skin-to-skin contact, with baby placed on mum's stomach or lower chest. No wrapping of baby. Father/companion joins in this bonding by placing hand on baby's back under warming blanket.

❏   Cord to be clamped and cut only after pulsation has ceased.

❏   That father/birth companion will cut cord after it stops pulsating.

❏   That father/companion/labour support be allowed to remain with mum in the operating and recovery room in the event of a C-section.

❏ That father will hold the baby after C-section birth and bring baby to mum for viewing and eye contact. In absence of urgency, father continues to hold baby for bonding.

❏ A wait for natural placenta delivery.

❏ Baby brought to breast to assist placenta birth.

❏ Gentle uterine massage every fifteen minutes to assist placenta birth.

❏ Natural nipple stimulation to assist in placenta expulsion.

❏ *No cord traction,* manual removal or use of Syntocinon for removal of placenta unless necessary.

❏ OTHER REQUESTS: ————————————————

FOR BABY

We request:

❏ To have bright lights temporarily removed at moment of birth and until baby is moved to mother's chest.

❏ Allow vernix to be absorbed into baby's skin; delay "cleaning or rubbing". Use of a *soft* cloth, not terry, when rubbing is appropriate.

❏ Baby to remain with mother and birth companion
   ❏ ½ hr.   ❏ 1 hr.   ❏ 2 hrs.

❏ Oral Vitamin K to be used rather than an injection if available.

❏ That father and baby stay with mother throughout the hospital stay.

❏ To have footprints made in the baby's birth book.

❏   Breastfeeding several times during the first few hours of baby's life.

❏   Breastfeeding only. No bottles, formula, pacifier or artificial nipples.

We thank you in advance for your support and kind attention to our choices. We know you join us in looking forward to a beautiful birth and celebration of this new life.

BIBLIOGRAPHY

BOOKS

Barber, Joseph, Ph.D., and Cheri Adrian, Ph.D., Eds. *Psychological Approaches to the Management of Pain.* Levittown, Pa.: Brunner/Mazel, 1982.

Barstow, Anne Llewellyn. *Witchcraze.* San Francisco: Pandora, 1994.

Bieler, Henry G., M.D. *Food Is Your Best Medicine.* New York: Random House, 1965.

Birch, William G., M.D. *A Doctor Discusses Pregnancy.* Chicago: Budlong Press, 1988.

Blaustone, Jan. *The Joy of Parenthood.* Deephaven, Minn.: Meadowbrook Press, 1993.

Bolduc, Henry Leo. *Self Hypnosis: Creating Your Own Destiny.* Independence, Va.: Adventures into Time Publishers, 1992.

Bradley, Robert A., M.D. *Husband-Coached Childbirth.* New York: Bantam Books, 1996.

Capacchione, Lucia, and Sandra Bardsley. *Creating a Joyful Birth Experience.* New York: Fireside, 1994.

Carola, Robert, et al. *Human Anatomy and Physiology.* New York: McGrawHill Education, 1990.

Carpenter, Carl. *Hypno Kinesiology: A Holistic Approach to Healing.* New Delhi, India: Sterling Publishers, 2003.

Chamberlain, David. *The Mind of Your Newborn Baby.* Berkeley, Calif.: North Atlantic Books, 1998.

Curtis, Glade B., and Judith Schuler. *Your Pregnancy Week by Week.* Cambridge, Mass.: DeCapo Press, 2004.

Davis, Elizabeth, et al. *Heart & Hands: A Midwife's Guide to Pregnancy and Birth.* Berkeley, Calif.: Celestial Arts, 2004.

Dick-Read, Grantly, M.D. *Childbirth Without Fear.* London: Pinter & Martin Ltd., 2004.

Dunham, Carroll, et al. *Mamatoto: A Celebration of Birth.* New York: Viking-Penguin, 1992.

Dye, John H., M.D. *Easy Childbirth: Healthy Mother and Healthy Children.* Buffalo, N.Y.: J. H. Dye Medical Institute, 1891.

Ehrenreich, Barbara, and Deirdre English. *Witches, Midwives and Nurses.* New York: The Feminist Press, 1972.

Ellerbe, Helen. *The Dark Side of Christian History.* Berkeley, Calif.: Morningstar Books, 1995.

Gaskin, Ina May. *Spiritual Midwifery.* Summertown, Tenn.: Book Publishing Co., 2002.

Goer, Henci. *The Thinking Woman's Guide to a Better Birth.* New York: Perigree Books, 1999.

Hawk, Breck, R.N., midwife. *Hey! Who's Having This Baby, Anyway?* Phoenix, Ariz.: End Table Books, 2005.

Harper, Barbara, R.N. *Gentle Birth Choices.* Rochester, Vt.: Healing Arts Press, 1994.

Hoke, James H. *I Would If I Could and I Can.* Glendale, Calif.: Westwood Publishing Co.. 1980.

Jones, Carl. *The Birth Partner's Handbook.* Deephaven, Minn.: Meadowbrook Press, 1989.

——. *Mind over Labor.* New York: Penguin Books, 1987.

Kerr, Mary Brandt. *The Joy of Pregnancy.* New York: Golden Apple Publishers, 1987.

Krasner, A.M., Ph.D. *The Wizard Within.* Irvine, Calif.: American Board of Hypnotherapy Press, 1990.

Kroger, William, M.D. *Childbirth with Hypnosis.* North Hollywood, Calif.: Wilshire Book Co., 1970.

Lazarev, Michael, M.D. *Sonatal.* Bloomsbury, N.J.: Infinite Potential, Inc., 1991.

Leboyer, Frederick. *Birth Without Violence.* Rochester, Vt.: Healing Arts Press, 2002.

Lennart, Righard. *Delivery Self-Attachment.* Sunland, Calif.: Geddes Productions, 1992.

Lesko, Wendy, and Matthew Lesko. *The Maternity Sourcebook.* New York: Warner Books, 1985.

Longacre, R.D., Ph.D., F.B.H.A. *Client-Centered Hypnotherapy.* Dubuque, Iowa: Kendall/Hunt Publishing Co., 1995.

Losier, Michael J. *Law of Attraction.* Victoria, B.C., Canada: Michael Losier, 2003.

McCutcheon, Susan. *Natural Childbirth the Bradley Way.* New York: Plume, 1996.

Mitford, Jessica. *The American Way of Birth.* New York: E. P. Dutton, 1992.

Nathanielsz, Peter, M.D. *The Prenatal Prescription.* New York: HarperCollins Publishers, 2001.

Northrup, Christiane, M.D., Ph.D. *Women's Bodies, Women's Wisdom.* New York: Bantam Books, 2002.

Odent, Michel, M.D. *Birth Reborn.* Medford, N.J.: Birth Works Press, 1994.

O'Toole, Marie T., Ed. *Miller-Keane Encyclopedia and Dictionary of Medicine, Nursing and Allied Health.* Philadelphia, Pa.: W. B. Saunders Co., 2003.

Peterson, Gayle, Ph.D. *An Easier Childbirth.* Berkeley, Calif.: Shadow and Light Publications, 1993.

Sears, William, M.D., and Martha Sears, R.N. *The Birth Book.* Boston, Mass.: Little, Brown, 1994.

Shanley, Laura Kaplan. *Unassisted Childbirth.* New York: Bergin & Garvey Paperback, 1994.

Simkin, Penny. *The Birth Partner.* Boston, Mass.: Harvard Common Press, 2001.

——, et al. *Pregnancy, Childbirth and the Newborn.* Deephaven, Minn.: Meadowbrook Press, 2001.

Stone, Merlin. *When God Was a Woman.* Orlando, Fla.: Harcourt Brace & Co., 1976.

Straus, Roger A., Ph.D. *Strategic Self-Hypnosis.* New York: Simon & Schuster, 2000.

Thomas, Clayton L., Ed. *Taber's Cyclopedic Medical Dictionary.* Philadelphia. Pa.: F. A. Davis Co., 1997.

Vander, Arthur, et al. *Human Physiology.* New York: McGraw-Hill Publishing Co., 1997.

Vaughn, Kathleen. *Safe Childbirth.* London: Bailliere, Tindall & Cox, 1937.

Verny, Thomas, M.D. *The Secret Life of the Unborn Child.* New York: Dell Publishing, 1981.

Weil, Andrew, M.D. *Spontaneous Healing.* New York: Ballantine Publishing Group, 1995.

Wessel, Helen. *The Joy of Natural Childbirth: Natural Childbirth and the Christian Family.* Santa Rosa Beach, Fla.: Bookmates International Inc., 1994.

Wildner, Kim. *Mother's Intention: How Belief Shapes Birth.* Ludington, Mich.: Harbor & Hill Publishing, 2003.

Wirth, Frederick, M.D. *Prenatal Parenting.* New York: HarperCollins Publishers, 2001.

BOOKLETS, ARTICLES, PERIODICALS AND RESEARCH

Carnation Health Care Services, *Pregnancy in Anatomical Illustrations*, Los Angeles, Calif., 1962.

Cesarean Prevention Movement, *Things You Can Do to Avoid an Unnecessary Cesarean*, Syracuse, N.Y., 1989.

"Childbirth Without Fear", *Life*, Jan. 1950.

Division of Maternal and Child Health, *Prenatal and Postnatal Care*, Dept. of Health & Human Services, Rockville, Md.

Gilman, Eleanor, "Turning Breech Babies with Hypnosis", *American Health*, Nov. 1995.

Kuhlman, Christine. "A Time for Letting Go", *Convergence Magazine*, 1989.

Levine, Beth, "Labor Intensive", *Woman's Day*, May 1996.

Mehl-Madronna, Louis, "Hypnosis and Conversion of the Breech to the Vertex Presentation", *Archives of Family Medicine*, Vol. 3, Oct. 1994.

Orr, Tamara B., "Controlling Pain through Hypnosis", *Back Pain Magazine*, May 1990.

Reed, Donna, *Goddess Remembered, The Burning Times, Full Circle*, National Film Board of Canada.

Ross Laboratories, *Becoming a Parent*, Ross Growth and Development Series, Columbus, Ohio, 1988.

Tow, Jennifer, "Labor Support, Empowering Women in Birth", *Spirit of Change Magazine*, Jan. 1998.

ABOUT THE AUTHOR

Marie (Mickey) Mongan, the former dean of a women's college, is the Director of the HypnoBirthing Institute, outside of Concord, New Hampshire. Mongan brings to her hypnotherapy and HypnoBirthing classrooms over thirty years of experience in education and counselling on the college level, and in the public and private sector. Early in her career, Mongan received recognition when she was named one of five outstanding New Hampshire educators and granted a Ford Foundation Fellowship to Harvard University.

She is licensed by the state of New Hampshire as a counsellor and holds certification as an advanced clinical hypnotherapist, a hypno-anaesthesiologist and an instructor of hypnotherapy. She holds many awards for achievement in the field of hypnotherapy, including the National Guild of Hypnotists President's Award, and the much-coveted Charles Tebbetts Award for her contribution to the understanding and acceptance of hypnotherapy within the medical field. She also is a recipient of the Plymouth State College Alumni Achievement Award.

In the spring of 1992, Mongan travelled to Moscow as an American Diplomat with the Bridges for Peace Foundation, where she taught personnel management techniques to Russian women.

Mickey Mongan is the mother of four adult children, all born with the Dick-Read method on which the HypnoBirthing philosophy is based. Her practice has included group and individual work in a wide spectrum of therapy applications, in addition to the HypnoBirthing programme that she shares with you in this book.

"This lively, highly readable little book is for everyone who works with maternity and neonatal services … a heartening, honest, practical, non-nonsense guide to a method of care that will appeal to most people for sensible reasons."
'*Infant Journal*'

Kangaroo Babies
Nathalie Charpak

£14.99

Kangaroo Mother Care was created to help premature and low-birth-weight-infants develop into healthy babies. The baby remains in direct skin-to-skin contact with its mother who provides, naturally, all the benefits of incubator care: the baby's body temperature is regulated, breastfeeding is stimulated, bonding is strengthened and the baby feels secure.

It is a natural approach to mothering, which will revolutionise the care of all newborn babies.

"We needed the well-documented book by Nathalie Charpak – an active member of the Kangaroo Foundation – to realize that the concept of marsupial babies is spreading at a high speed all over the world." *Michel Odent, author of 'Birth Reborn'*

Infant Massage
Vimala McClure

£9.99

Master the techniques of infant massage so that you incorporate this wonderful healing art into your baby's life. Vimala McClure shows how a daily massage can be one of the greatest gifts a child can receive, bringing physical and psychological benefits to both parents and babies.

Massage benefits babies – easing discomfort; releasing tension; helping premature babies to gain weight; relief of colic, fever, chest and nasal congestion – as well as bonding the baby to its parents.

Birth Reborn
Michel Odent

£12.99

For over 40 years Michel Odent has been the world's leading 'birth guru'. He has pioneered a new philosophy of childbirth, making it a natural experience for women and providing settings that allow a woman to give birth her own way. Women become their own birthing experts, if they follow their instincts they can birth naturally, with the minimal intervention of medical science.

Birth Reborn gives expectant mothers the confidence and information they need in order to trust themselves to give birth without the drugs and medical procedures that are being increasingly recognised as harmful to the mother and to the baby's future development.